Alkaloids - Their Importance in Nature and Human Life

Edited by Joanna Kurek

Published in London, United Kingdom

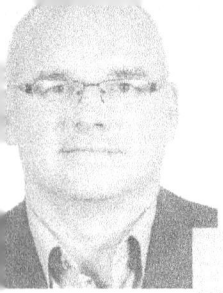
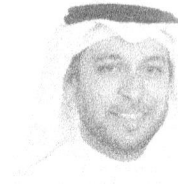
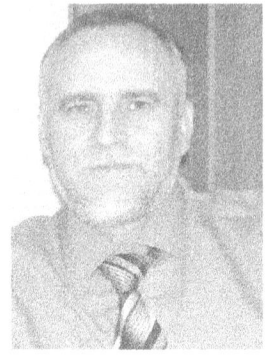
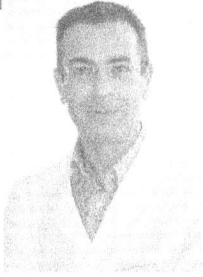
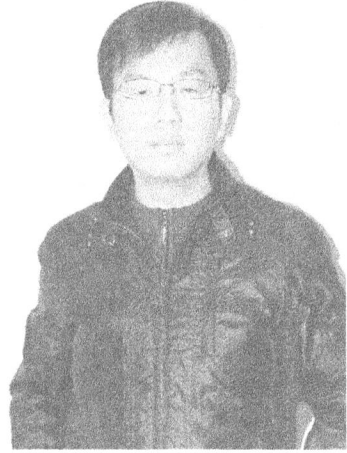
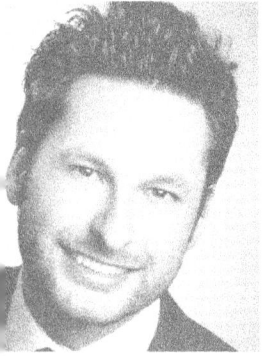
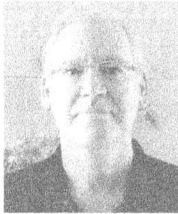

IntechOpen

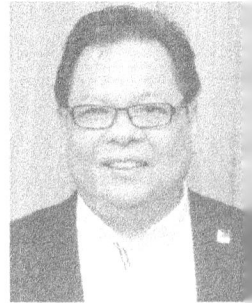
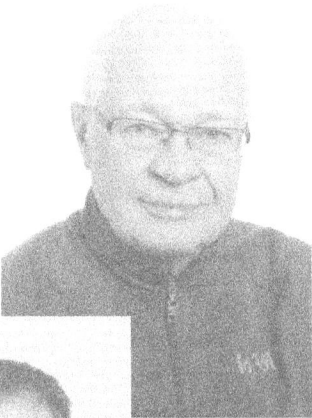
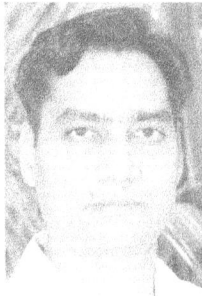
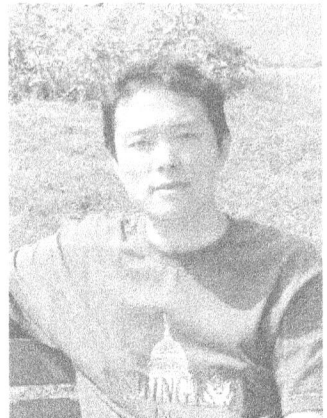
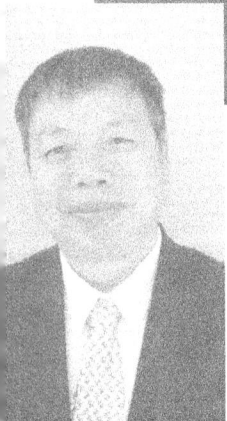
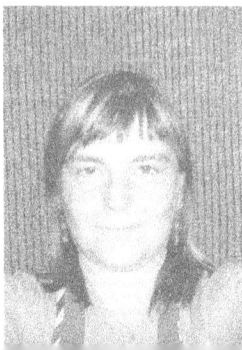

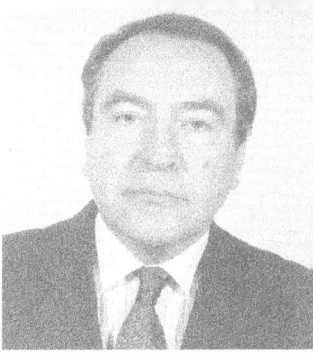

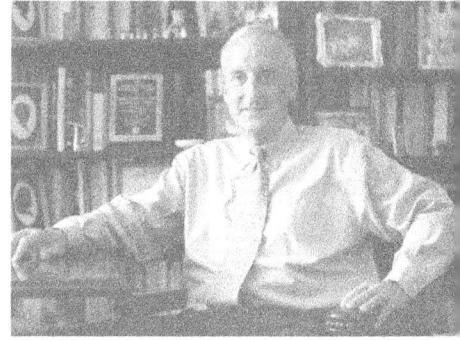

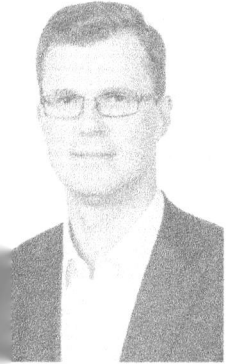

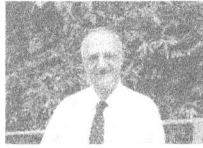

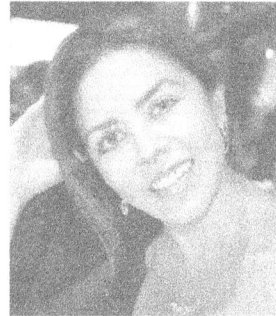

Supporting open minds since 2005

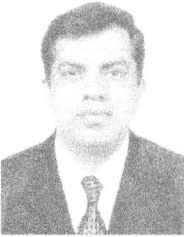

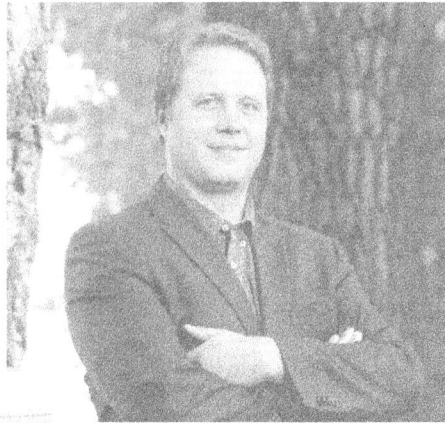

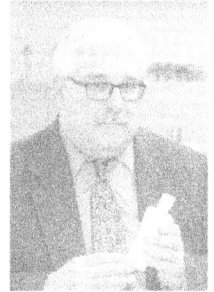

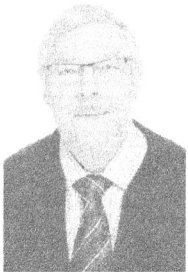

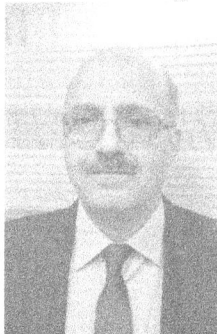

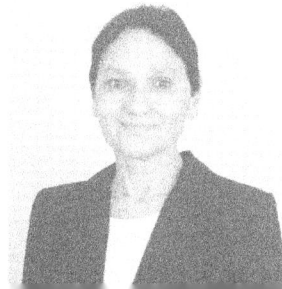

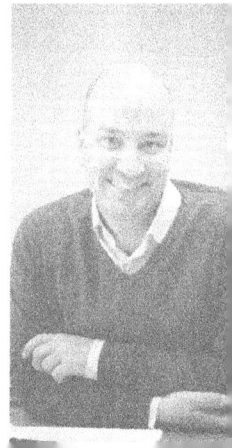

Alkaloids - Their Importance in Nature and Human Life
http://dx.doi.org/10.5772/intechopen.73336
Edited by Joanna Kurek

Contributors
Abdulmajeed Alsamarrai, Hebert Jair Barrales-Cureño, Adrián Gómez De Jesús, Juan Antonio Cortés Ruíz, Jesús Antonio Salazar Magallón, Jorge Montiel Montoya, Leticia Mónica Sánchez Herrera, Maria Carmina Calderón Caballero, Luis Germán López Valdez, César Reyes Reyes, Jose Espinoza-Perez, Irma Vásquez García, Nigel Brunton, Md Abu Bakar Siddique, Weiwei Zhang, Huijing Li, Yan-Chao Wu, Joanna Kurek

Notice
Statements and opinions expressed in the chapters are these of the individual contributors and not necessarily those of the editors or publisher. No responsibility is accepted for the accuracy of information contained in the published chapters. The publisher assumes no responsibility for any damage or injury to persons or property arising out of the use of any materials, instructions, methods or ideas contained in the book.

First published in London, United Kingdom, 2019 by IntechOpen
IntechOpen is the global imprint of INTECHOPEN LIMITED, registered in England and Wales, registration number: 11086078, 7th floor, 10 Lower Thames Street, London, EC3R 6AF, United Kingdom
Printed in Croatia

British Library Cataloguing-in-Publication Data
A catalogue record for this book is available from the British Library

Additional hard and PDF copies can be obtained from orders@intechopen.com

Alkaloids - Their Importance in Nature and Human Life
Edited by Joanna Kurek
p. cm.
Print ISBN 978-1-78984-576-1
Online ISBN 978-1-78984-577-8
eBook (PDF) ISBN 978-1-78984-692-8

We are IntechOpen,
the world's leading publisher of
Open Access books
Built by scientists, for scientists

4,300+
Open access books available

117,000+
International authors and editors

130M+
Downloads

151
Countries delivered to

Our authors are among the
Top 1%
most cited scientists

12.2%
Contributors from top 500 universities

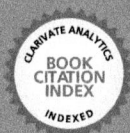

Interested in publishing with us?
Contact book.department@intechopen.com

Numbers displayed above are based on latest data collected.
For more information visit www.intechopen.com

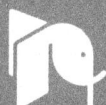

Meet the editor

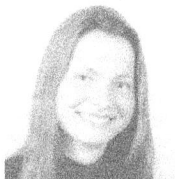

Joanna Kurek is a doctor of chemistry at the Faculty of Chemistry at Adam Mickiewicz University in Poznań, Poland, and is currently working in the Laboratory for Chemistry of Heterocyclic Compounds in the Chemistry Department at the same university. She studied chemistry and received her master's degree in Chemistry from Adam Mickiewicz University. She is interested in organic chemistry and natural compounds, especially alkaloids. Currently, her scientific interests are alkaloids, especially colchicine, its various derivatives, and their biological activities.

Contents

Preface

Alkaloids are a vast group of naturally occurring organic compounds. They are mainly produced by certain plant species rather than by animals and are secondary metabolites. For thousands of years, they have been indispensable in the human diet in the form of food and drinks and were also especially useful as medicines. Alkaloids are very active compounds and induce specific reactions in the human body. They are antimitotic, anti-inflammatory, anticancer, antibacterial, analgesic, local anesthetic and pain relief, neuropharmacological, antimicrobial, antifungal, anticorrosive, antiplasmodic, antiparasitic, antioxidative, antibacterial, anti-HIV, and insecticidal agents. Nowadays, scientists are trying to discover new semisynthetic and synthetic derivatives of naturally occurring alkaloids that will be effective medicines and also could possess new applications.

This book contains chapters that describe various alkaloid applications. The chapters are written by scientists who are specialized in this field.

I wish to thank Martina Josavac and Danijela Sakic, Author Service Managers at IntechOpen, for all email correspondence, which made this book possible.

Joanna Kurek
Chemistry Department,
Adam Mickiewicz University in Poznań,
Poland

Chapter 1

Introductory Chapter: Alkaloids - Their Importance in Nature and for Human Life

Joanna Kurek

1. Introduction

In nature there are many natural compounds. From among many classes of naturally occurring organic compounds such as carbohydrates, lipids, proteins, amino acids, anthocyanins, flavonoids, and steroids, the one that seems to be quite special is alkaloids. What makes them special? They derived from amino acids and can be synthetized as secondary metabolites by plants and some animals. These compounds play an important role in living organisms. Alkaloids occurred to be extremely important for human beings for ages, besides they are secondary metabolites, what could suggest that they are useless. Alkaloids showed strong biological effects on animal and human organisms in very small doses. Alkaloids are present not only in human daily life in food and drinks but also as stimulant drugs. They showed anti-inflammatory, anticancer, analgesics, local anesthetic and pain relief, neuropharmacologic, antimicrobial, antifungal, and many other activities. Alkaloids are useful as diet ingredients, supplements, and pharmaceuticals, in medicine and in other applications in human life. Alkaloids are also important compounds in organic synthesis for searching new semisynthetic and synthetic compounds with possibly better biological activity than parent compounds.

2. About alkaloids

Alkaloids are a huge group of naturally occurring organic compounds which contain nitrogen atom or atoms (amino or amido in some cases) in their structures. These nitrogen atoms cause alkalinity of these compounds. These nitrogen atoms are usually situated in some ring (cyclic) system. For example, indole alkaloids are those that contain nitrogen atom in indole ring system. Generally based on structures, alkaloids can be divided into classes like indoles, quinolines, isoquinolines, pyrrolidines, pyridines, pyrrolizidines, tropanes, and terpenoids and steroids. Other classification system is connected with a family of plant species that they occur. One of the examples is the opium alkaloids that occur in the opium poppy (*Papaver somniferum*) [1]. These two different classification systems cause confusion between their biological distribution and the chemical types of alkaloids, because there is not unmistakable correlation.

Alkaloids (whose name originally comes from "alkali-like") can react with acids and then form salts, just like inorganic alkalis. These nitrogen atoms can behave like a base in acid-base reactions. In general alkaloids, which are treated as amines, the same as amines in their names, have suffix -ine. Alkaloids in pure form are usually colorless, odorless crystalline solids, but sometimes they can be yellowish liquids. Quite often, they have bitter taste. Now more than 3000 of alkaloids are known in over different 4000 plant species.

These compounds are produced generally by many plant species, mainly by flowering plants and also by some animals. Plants produce and store many organic compounds like amino acids, proteins, carbohydrates, fats, and alkaloids, which are usually treated as secondary metabolites. They are stored in each part of the plant—leaves, stem, root, and fruits of plants—but in different amounts. It was suggested that they are plants' waste product, but now evidence suggests that they play some important biological function in plants.

Some groups of structurally related alkaloids are present in plants from few to even 30. These alkaloids belong to the same class but have some differences in their structure and one of them usually occurs in majority. Some plant families are very rich in alkaloids. For example, in plants like opium poppy (*Papaver somniferum*) and the ergot fungus (*Claviceps*), there are about 30 different alkaloid types. In plants, their function is still mostly unknown. Alkaloids because of their bitter taste are natural compound to deter herbivorous organisms. In some plants they are used as natural pesticides. It was suggested that alkaloids in plants have a function to protect them from destructive activity of some insect species. Alkaloids are also present in some animal species like frogs (poison dart frogs (*Phyllobates*)), New World beaver (*Castor canadensis*), and lizards, and they are produced by fungi species and ergot.

Besides having the same general name—alkaloids—they have an extreme variety of chemical structures. Some of these compounds seem to have people known for ages because of their wide range of activity on human organisms and also other animals. For thousand years, extracts from plants containing alkaloids had medicinal use as drugs, and they owe their powerful effects thanks to the presence of alkaloids. Morphine was the first alkaloid which was isolated about 1804 from opium poppy in crystalline form. Alkaloids are an interesting group of compounds with a wide range of activities, undesirable and desirable, on animal and human organisms. Alkaloids have diverse physiological effects: antibacterial, antimitotic, anti-inflammatory, analgesic, local anesthetic, hypnotic, psychotropic, and antitumor activity and many others. Nowadays, alkaloids usually from plants rather than from animals are still of great interest to organic chemists, biologists, biochemists, pharmacologists, and pharmacists. Well-known alkaloids include morphine, strychnine, quinine, atropine, caffeine, ephedrine, and nicotine [1].

3. Methods of isolation

Extracts of plants containing alkaloids were known and used because of their diverse activity by people from ages. But ages ago people did not know direct methods to isolate pure compounds from specified plant species. Alkaloids in plants usually exist as aqueous solution in tissues. To isolate them the method called extraction is usually used. For commercially useful alkaloids, special extraction methods were developed. In general mixture containing alkaloid should be dissolved with some solvent with reagents. Extraction method allows recovery of alkaloids from solution. Then, each alkaloid can be separated from mixture and be obtained in pure form. To obtain crystalline form of alkaloids, certain solvents should be used. Another method is chromatography. It uses differences in degrees of adsorption of different alkaloids in some solvent system on solid materials such as silica or alumina.

4. Pharmaceutical and medicinal use of alkaloids

Alkaloids showed quite diverse medicinal properties. Many of them possess local anesthetic properties, but their practical use is limited for clinical purpose. Morphine (**Figure 1a**) is one of the most known alkaloids which had been used and still is for medical purposes. This alkaloid is a powerful narcotic which is used for the relief of pain, but its usefulness is limited because of addictive properties [1].

Methyl ether derivative of morphine—codeine—naturally occurring next to morphine in the opium poppy, possesses an excellent analgesic activity and is shown to be relatively nonaddictive. These alkaloids act as respiratory or cardiac stimulants. Next, the alkaloid which is used as medication in many clinical applications is atropine (**Figure 1b**). For example, injection with atropine is given to treat bradycardia (low heart rate).

Tubocurarine (**Figure 2**) is an alkaloid, is an ingredient of poison curare, and is used in surgery as muscle relaxant. Alkaloids vincristine and vinblastine are used as chemotherapeutic agent in the treatment of many cancer types. Cocaine an alkaloid present in *Erythroxylum coca* is a potent local anesthetic. Ergonovine, an alkaloid from the fungus *Claviceps purpurea*, and the second alkaloid ephedrine isolated from *Ephedra* species both act as blood vessel constrictors. Also ephedrine is used in bronchial asthma and to relieve discomfort of hay fever, sinusitis, and common colds.

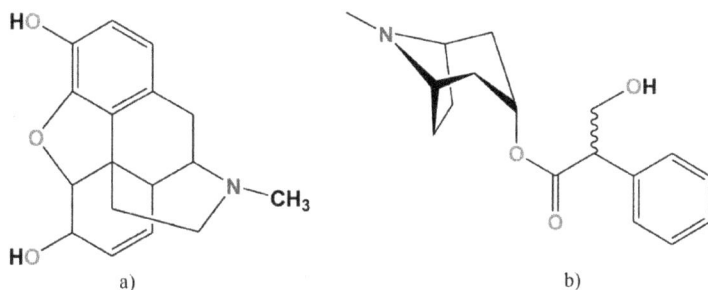

Figure 1.
Structures of alkaloids: (a) morphine and (b) atropine.

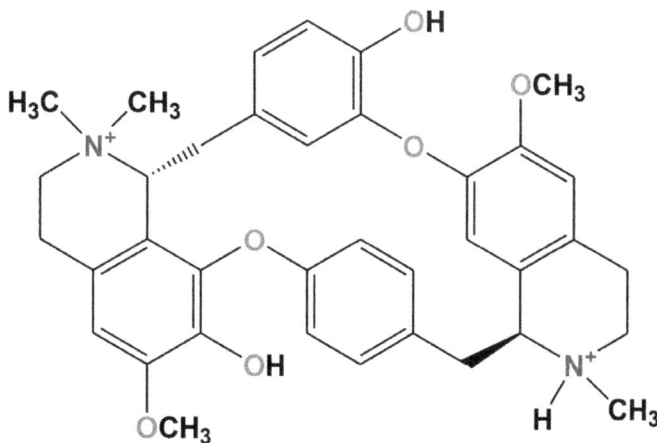

Figure 2.
Structure of tubocurarine.

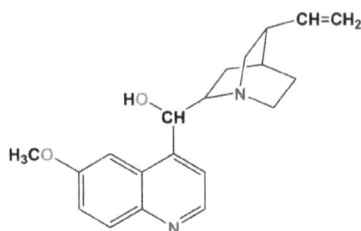

Figure 3.
Structure of quinine from Cinchona species.

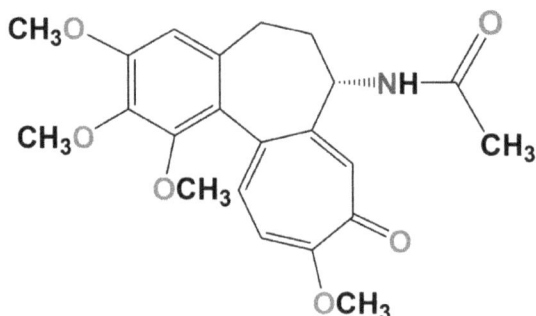

Figure 4.
Structure of colchicine.

Quinine (**Figure 3**) is a powerful antimalarial agent and more often is replaced by synthetic drugs, which are more effective and less toxic. Another alkaloid from *Cinchona* species is quinidine which has medical application as treatment of irregular rhythms of the heartbeat or arrhythmias.

Colchicine (**Figure 4**) is another alkaloid, present in plants of Liliaceae family, known for ages to treat acute gout attacks. Another clinically used alkaloid is lobeline isolated from *Lobelia inflata*, which has multiple mechanisms of action.

5. Alkaloids in human food and drinks

Many alkaloids are elements of human diet, both in food and drinks. The plants in the human diet in which alkaloids are present are not only coffee seeds (caffeine, **Figure 5**), cacao seeds (theobromine and caffeine), and tea leaves (theophylline,

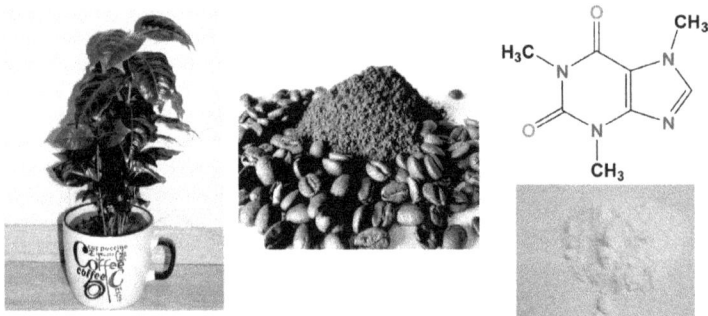

Figure 5.
Plant source of caffeine and its structure and powdered caffeine (pure form) (author's own photos).

caffeine) but also tomatoes (tomatine) and potatoes (solanine). The most common alkaloid is caffeine which has also application as an ingredient of soft drinks like Coca-Cola to improve their taste and in drinks for active people who do sport.

Other known alkaloid with bitter taste used as an ingredient of tonics is quinine (**Figure 3**) isolated from *Cinchona* species.

6. Alkaloids as stimulants

Alkaloids stimulate human organisms, for example, central nervous system, or directly work on the human brain. Nicotine (**Figure 6**) is an alkaloid obtained from the tobacco plant (*Nicotiana tabacum*) and is a potent stimulant and the main ingredient in tobacco smoked in pipes, cigars, and cigarettes. This alkaloid is highly addictive [1].

Cocaine is a narcotic drug, which activity is not suitable for medical purposes. This alkaloid has an opposite effect than morphine. This compound produces in the human body a euphoric hyperarousal state, but high doses of it may lead to fibrillation and death.

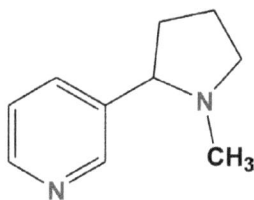

Figure 6.
Structure of nicotine.

7. Dark nature of alkaloids

Some alkaloids are illicit drugs and poisons. Poisonous activities of some alkaloids are known for ages. One of these is strychnine (from *Strychnos* species, **Figure 7**). One of the well-known poison curare (obtained from *Chondrodendron tomentosum*) used in the South Africa as narrow poison contains alkaloid tubocurarine.

Coniine is an alkaloid isolated from *Conium maculatum*, which is an active ingredient of poison hemlock. Mescaline isolated from *Anhalonium* species has hallucinogenic activity. Psilocybin is a naturally occurring drug isolated from fungi species *Psilocybe mexicana* and possesses psychedelic activity. During the past

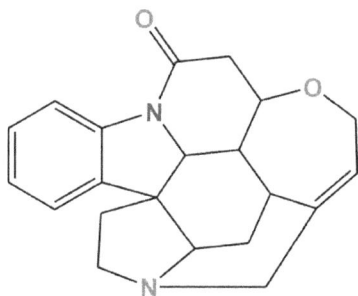

Figure 7.
Structure of strychnine.

decades, many semisynthetic derivatives of naturally occurring alkaloids with various activities have been synthesized. Synthetic derivative of morphine is heroin, and, from lysergic acid naturally present in *C. purpurea*, LSD was produced.

8. Other practical use of alkaloids

Besides activities mentioned above, alkaloids from many different plant species have many other useful applications such as antiparasitic [2], antiplasmodial [3], anticorrosive [4], antioxidative [5], antibacterial [6], anti-HIV [7], and insecticidal activities [8].

9. Conclusion

Alkaloids are very important compounds for human beings. For ages their extracts were used as a cure to rescue people from pain like morphine and some illnesses like quinine in malaria and colchicine in gout. Thanks to alkaloids during ages, people can cure the diseases and improve their life.

Scientists still keep trying to design and synthetize more and more semisynthetic and synthetic alkaloids derived from natural sources of alkaloids. These alkaloids possibly can possess interesting activities for medical, pharmaceutical, synthetic, and many other useful properties.

Author details

Joanna Kurek
Chemistry Department, Adam Mickiewicz University, Poznań, Poland

*Address all correspondence to: joankur@amu.edu.pl

IntechOpen

References

[1] Chisholm H. Encyclopedia Brittanica, A Dictionary of Arts, Sciences, Literature and General Information. Vol. 22. New York: Sagwan Press; 2015. ISBN-13: 9781340141998. https://www.britannica.com

[2] Fernandez LS, Sykes ML, Andrews KT, Avery VM. Antiparasitic activity of alkaloids from plant species of Papua New Guinea and Australia. International Journal of Antimicrobial Agents. 2010;**36**(3):275-279. DOI: 10.1016/j.ijantimicag.2010.05.008

[3] Frédérich M, Jacquier MJ, Thépenier P, De Mol P, Tits M, Philippe G, et al. Antiplasmodial activity of alkaloids from various *Strychnos* species. Journal of Natural Products. 2002;**65**(10):1381-1386. DOI: 10.1021/np020070e

[4] Capasso A, Aquino R, De Tommasi N, Piacente S, Rastrelli L, Pizza C. Neuropharmacology activity of alkaloids from South American medicinal plants. Current Medicinal Chemistry: Central Nervous System Agents. 2002;**2**(1):1-15. DOI: 10.2174/1568015024606600

[5] Czapski GA, Szypuła W, Kudlik M, Wileńska B, Kania M, Danikiewicz W, et al. Assessment of antioxidative activity of alkaloids from *Huperzia selago* and *Diphasiastrum complanatum* using in vitro systems. Folia Neuropathologica. 2014;**52**(4):394-406. DOI: 10.5114/fn.2014.47840

[6] Karou D, Savadogo A, Canini A, Yameogo S, Montesano C, Simpore J, et al. Antibacterial activity of alkaloids from *Sida acuta*. African Journal of Biotechnology. 2005;**4**(12):1452-1457

[7] Zhang H, Zhang C-R, Shan Han Y, Wainberg MA, Yue J-M. New *Securinega* alkaloids with anti-HIV activity from *Flueggea virosa*. RSC Advances. 2015;**5**(129):107045-107053. DOI: 10.1039/C5RA22191A

[8] Ge Y, Liu P, Yang R, Zhang L, Chen H, Camara I, et al. Insecticidal constituents and activity of alkaloids from *Cynanchum mongolicum*. Molecules. 2015;**20**:17483-17492. DOI: 10.3390/molecules200917483

Chapter 2

Alkaloids of Pharmacological Importance in *Catharanthus roseus*

Hebert Jair Barrales-Cureño, César Reyes Reyes,

Irma Vásquez García, Luis Germán López Valdez,

Adrián Gómez De Jesús, Juan Antonio Cortés Ruíz,

Leticia Mónica Sánchez Herrera,

María Carmina Calderón Caballero,

Jesús Antonio Salazar Magallón, Jose Espinoza Perez

and Jorge Montiel Montoya

Abstract

Catharanthus roseus is a plant of the *Apocynaceae* family. It produces over 120 alkaloids, 70 of which are pharmacologically active. *C. roseus* produces vinblastine, utilized in treating Hodgkin's disease; testicular tumors, breast carcinoma, chorio-carcinoma, Kaposi sarcoma and Letterer-Siwe disorder. Vincristine is used to treat acute lymphocytic leukemia, lymphosarcoma, lympho-granulomatosis and in solid infant tumors. The preparation process of 1 kg of vincristine has a cost of US\$ 3.5 million, while vinblastine has a cost of US\$1 million. Therefore, 530 kg of dry leaves are necessary to produce 1 kg of vincristine and half a ton for getting 1 g of vinblastine. The high cost is due to the low concentrations in the aerial portion. Due to the high market value and its effectiveness in different medical treatments, this chapter deals with the pharmacological application of the *C. roseus* alkaloids.

Keywords: antileukemic, indole-monoterpene alkaloids, Letterer-Siwe disorder, vinblastine, vincristine

1. Introduction

Catharanthus roseus (L.) G. Don is a medicinal plant of the *Apocynaceae* family, originally from Madagascar. In the present, it has been naturalized in all tropical regions of the world. *C. roseus* produces 120 alkaloids, 70 of which have pharmaco-logical activity, for example, vindosine, hörhammericine, lochnericine, vindolicine, anhydrovinblastine, vincristine, tabersonine, catharanthine, vindoline, yohimbine, vinblastine, ajmalicine. Terpenoid indole alkaloids (TIA) are specially cultivated in an industrial scale to obtain anticancer alkaloids for the pharmaceutical industry [1]. The market of its leaves is monopolized by the United States and countries of Eastern Europe, like Hungary. In addition, attempts to obtain these alkaloids by *in vitro* tissue culture (cells in suspension) have not been very promising, since there are many yet unknown enzymes involved in their biosynthesis. *C. roseus* alkaloids isolated from leaf, root, and flower can be analyzed through chemical, chromatographic, and spectroscopic analytical methods. It has been estimated that active alkaloid content in leaves is very low—2 tons of leaves are needed to isolate and purify 1 g of vincristine, the amount needed for the treatment of an infant during 6 weeks. Vinblastine and vincristine alkaloids are potent chemotherapeutics with anticancer activity [2–5], and they also have tumor inhibition properties for the treatment of leukemia [6], lymphosarcoma (cancer in the lymphogenous system), lymphogranulomatosis (cancer in cervical lymphatic ganglia) and other malign tumors. Vinblastine is used in the treatment of Hodgkin's disease (it has a ganglion onset and it extends initially through the lymphatic system and later through the blood) the diagnosis must be made when typical Reed-Sternberg cells are found [7–9]. Letterer-Siwe disease (the average age for this disease is 2 years; it is a generally acute and disseminated dermatosis, which is characterized by lesions simulating seborrhoeic dermatitis distributed in hairy skin, neck, and trunk. The presence of purple papules, pustules, vesicles, and petechiae, and also systemic signs that include fever, anemia, lymphadenopathies, osteolytic lesions, and hepatosplenomegaly, has been described) [10]. It is effective in the treatment of advance testicular tumors, breast carcinoma, choriocarcinoma (malign neoplasy originated form the gestational trophoblast, of great aggressivity when not treated at the right time [11]. Kaposi's sarcoma (mesenchymatous tumor with the involvement of blood and lymphatic vessels, originated by the human herpesvirus 8, also known as Kaposi's sarcoma-associated herpesvirus [12], while drugs with hypotensor effect are prepared with ajmalicine and reserpine [13, 14]. These alkaloids are produced and accumulated exclusively in *C. roseus* plants, and only in trace amounts, around 0.0005% of the dry weight, which makes their extraction hard and costly. According to Loyola-Vargas and colleagues, the process for extracting 1 kg of vinblastine costs 1 million dollars, while 3.5 million are needed to produce the same amount of vincristine [15]. The high cost of these substances is due to them being found in very low concentrations in the aerial part of the plant (around 0.0005% of dry weight); which is why half a ton of dry leaves of *C. roseus* are needed for the obtention of 1 g of vinblastine [16] while to produce 1 kg of vincristine 530 kg are used [17]. Besides, their extraction is very complicated since it is carried out in the presence of 200 molecules with similar chemical and physical properties. The low production of vinblastine and vincristine, the high value in the market, and their effectiveness in different medical treatments have fostered research to determine their biosynthesis and to develop alternate production methods [18]. The production of vinblastine and vincristine has recently been induced and studied in *in vitro* cultures of plant tissues through hormone combinations of auxins and cytokinins [1]. Plant tissue *in vitro* culture biotechnology is a successful tool for the productive generation of calli and cells that produce secondary metabolites of pharmaceutical and medical importance, such as the alkaloids vincristine and vinblastine from *Catharanthus roseus* [18]. The objectives of this chapter emphasize and point out the main pharmacological applications of the species *Catharanthus roseus*. Its phenotype, biological action mechanism, biosynthesis of terpenoid indole alkaloids, and alkaloid extraction, analysis and production in *in vitro* cultures of *C. roseus* are described.

2. Phenotypic characteristics of *Catharanthus roseus*

C. roseus is an annual herb, woody in its base and ramified, it measures 80 cm in height. It has well developed roots and it flowers all year long, which is why it is used as an ornamental plant. Its leaves are opposite, oblong, with round apex, simple, whole, dark green color, shiny in the upper side, and of short petioles. Its branches can be erect or decumbent, and its relatively big flowers are axillary, solitary, of short peduncle and with five petals. Its fruit is a dehiscent follicle that contains numerous seeds (more than 20) of color black [19, 20]. There are several forms differentiated by flower coloration, probably due to genotypic variations, prevailing those of white color, white with red centre, red centre, dark rose (almost purple), white with disperse centre to violet rose or with dark centre bordered with red. This species of wild plant can tolerate many types of biotic and abiotic stress.

3. Mechanism of biological action

Vincristine and vinblastine are potent mitotic inhibitors used in leukemia chemotherapy; they are structures hard to synthesize chemically, like other cancer-fighting drugs such as taxol [21] thus biotechnological approaches represent the best route for its obtention. Vincristine binds to the tubulin β-subunit, the precursor protein of microtubules responsible of mitosis and other essential cellular functions like substrate transport, cellular mobility, and structural integrity, and it inhibits microtubule formation—this disruption causes cellular death and mitosis arrest [22].

4. Biosynthesis of terpenoid indole alkaloids of *Catharanthus roseus*

It has been shown that the biosynthesis of terpenoid indole alkaloids (TIA) in *C. roseus* is subject to strict control at the level of cells, tissues, and organs—in addition, it depends to a great extent on the own developmental stages of the plant and the surrounding environment. Several studies have dealt with the regulation of some of the genes coding for the enzymes involved in the synthesis of TIA and recently some of the molecular mechanisms controlling gene expression in cell suspension cultures of *C. roseus* have been elucidated [23]. The first step in TIA biosynthesis is the formation of tryptamine [24] from the L-tryptophane amino acid in a reaction catalyzed by the TDC enzyme. This cytosolic enzyme binds the primary metabolism with the secondary metabolism and its activity is considered as a limiting step, although not the only one, in the control of TIA biosynthesis [25]. Another limiting step in the biosynthesis is the tryptamine that binds to the secologanin monoterpene, the final product of the biosynthetic route of iridoids, in a reaction catalyzed by the STR1 enzyme. Tryptamine condensation with iridoid glucoside secologanin under the catalysis of the strictosidine synthase (STR) results in the formation of strictosidine, the central intermediary in the biosynthesis of all types of indole alkaloids [26]. Subsequently, strictosidine is metabolized through different enzymatic steps, including those catalyzed by D4H and DAT enzymes that lead to the formation of vindoline and catharanthine, the monoterpene alkaloids precursors to vinblastine and vincristine [27]. The main alkaloids obtained from *C. roseus* are shown in **Figure 1**: (1) vindolicine; (2) anhydrovinblastine; (3) vincristine; (4) ajmalicine; (5) tabersonine; (6) catharanthine; (7) vindoline; (8) vinblastine; and (9) ajmalicine.

4.1 Vindoline formation

Strictosidine β-D-glucosidase (SGD) is the enzyme that performs an important role in guiding monoterpenoid indole alkaloids biosynthesis in a specific direction.

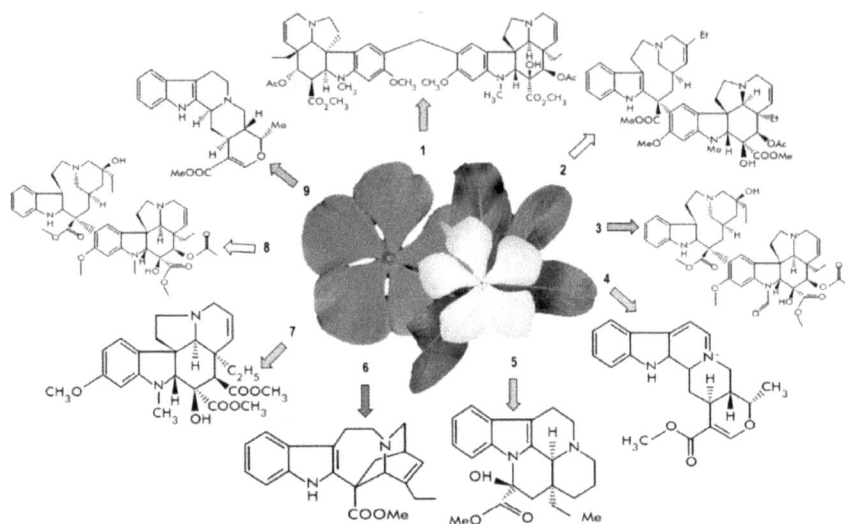

Figure 1.
Alkaloids produced by Catharanthus roseus (1) vindolicine ($C_{51}H_{64}N_4O_{12}$, 925.08 g/mol);
(2) anhydrovinblastine ($C_{46}H_{56}N_4O_8$, 792.97 g/mol); (3) vincristine ($C_{46}H_{56}N_4O_{10}$, 824.95 g/mol);
(4) ajmalicine ($C_{21}H_{24}N_2O_3$, 352.43 g/mol); (5) tabersonine ($C_{21}H_{24}N_2O_2$, 336.44 g/mol); (6)
catharanthine ($C_{21}H_{24}N_2O_2$, 336.42); (7) vindoline ($C_{25}H_{32}N_2O_6$, 456.53 g/mol); (8) vinblastine
($C_{46}H_{58}N_4O_9$, 810.97 g/mol); and (9) ajmalicine ($C_{21}H_{24}N_2O_3$, 352.43 g/mol).

The elimination of the rest of the glucose of strictosidine by SGD leads to an unstable, highly reactive aglucone, that is believed to convert into 4,21 dehydrogeissoschizine. It is believed that the latter is converted into cathenamine by the cathenamine synthase. Cathenamine is then converted into tabersonine through several steps, transforming into vindoline by a six-step sequence [28].

4.2 Regulation of tdc, str-1, d4h, and dat genes in *Catharanthus roseus*

Gene and enzyme regulation participating in TIA biosynthesis in *C. roseus* depends on the biological system employed, i.e., it differs from cell cultures to plants and within these it depends on the tissue and developmental stages analyzed. In addition, it has been found that the molecular mechanisms of regulation respond differentially to the presence of elicitors or to conditions of light and hormone stress, among others [29].

4.3 tdc and str1 genes

In *C. roseus* plants, high levels of mRNA for tdc and str1 have been observed in roots and leaves, the latter induced by UV light. The tdc and str1 transcripts and their respective proteins show high cellular and tissue specificity, for example, they have been detected exclusively in the superior and inferior epidermis of leaves, in stem epidermis, and flower buds [30].

In cell cultures of *C. roseus*, tdc and str1 are highly regulated at the transcriptional level. The expression of these two genes is inhibited by the presence of auxins, although they are induced by elicitation with fungi, yeast extraction, methyl jasmonate (MeJa), salicylic acid, and chitosan. These results suggest that the expression of str1 and tdc in cell cultures of *C. roseus* is regulated in a coordinated way by similar molecular mechanisms. The presence of some elements responding to elicitation in the promoter of the tdc gene has been determined. The architectural analysis of this promoter using tdc-gusA fusions in transgenic tobacco showed that the region between the positions −538 and −112 is determinant to control expression levels in different plant organs [31]. In addition, three functional regions of this promoter were identified starting from the position −160. A region between positions −160 and −99 increased transcription, and two regions, one between −99 and −87, and the other one between −87 and −37, responded differently to elicitation. To determine the regulatory mechanisms of str1, progressive deletions in the 5′ region of str1 promoter were joined to the reporter gene 3-glucuroni-dase (gusA) and their studied activity in transgenic tobacco. The analysis of the promoter of the str1 gene of *C. roseus* showed that the activator sequences are located between the positions −339 and −145. In other experiments, [32] showed that the biosynthetic route of jasmonate (octadecanoic acid pathway) was an integral part of the signal transduction pathway leading to the expression of tdc and str1 genes in cells in suspension of *C. roseus*.

The expression of the promoter of the gene str1 in transgenic cellular cultures of *C. roseus*, transformed with a construction containing the fusion str1/gusA, showed that a fraction of str1 promoter located in the position −369 is sufficient to induce the expression of the gusA gene in response to MeJa. In a subsequent report, [33] identified an element of 42 base pairs (pb) within the 396 pb fragment—the Jasmonate and Elicitor Responsive Element (JERE). The JERE region showed a GCC sequence in the str1 promoter that was necessary and sufficient for gene expression in the treatment with elicitors and jasmonate. Using the hybridization system of double hybrids and the JERE region as "bait", two cDNA coding for ORCA proteins (Octadecanoic derivative Responsive Catharanthus AP2-domain) were isolated. The AP2 domain is found exclusively in plant transcription factors and is involved in the regulation of several stress responses. In cell suspension cultures of *C. roseus*, str1 expression due to the jasmonate effect is mediated by the ORCA2 protein. Also, expression of the ORCA2 transcript was induced by elicitors, including yeast extract and MeJa. Recently, a new transcription factor (ORCA3) was discovered in cell suspension cultures of *C. roseus*. ORCA3 coordinately regulates multiple genes, including dxs, tdc, str1, sgd, cpr, and d4h, which code for pathway routes both of primary and secondary metabolism related to TIA formation [23].

4.4 d4h and dat genes

In *C. roseus* plantlings, d4h is induced by the presence of light and their transcription levels are increased after treatment with MeJa [34]. *In situ* hybridization and immunolocalization studies have showed that d4h and its protein are located in specialized cells (laticifers and idioblasts) shown in young leaves, stems and flower buds of *C. roseus* [30]. Both the transcripts of dat gene and its protein are co-located with d4h and D4H in laticifers and idioblasts [30]. In addition, studies with intact plants and with plantlings have shown that the induction of the mRNA of dat, and DAT activity and accumulation occur preferentially in leaves and cotyledons of etiolated plants treated with light, but they are not present in roots nor in cell suspension cultures, which explains the impossibility of producing vinblastine and vincristine in cell systems.

5. Pharmacological application of *Catharanthus roseus* alkaloids

5.1 Clinical pharmacology

Vinblastine is a drug used in the elective regime for the metastatic treatment of testicular cancer. The estimates of half-life after vinblastine administration to patients were 4 min, 1.6 h, and 25 h, which indicates a faster drug distribution in most tissues and a subsequent slower terminal elimination process. Distribution and initial cleaning phase for vincristine are kinetically comparable to the ones observed for vinblastine; half-lives for those phases have been reported at 4 min and 2.3 h in studies with vincristine. The terminal elimination phase for vincristine is reported to be three to four times longer than the one estimated for vinblastine, and the slow elimination of vincristine from the neuronal susceptible tissue suggest that it plays a role in neurotoxicity commonly seen in clinical adjustments with vincristine but not with vinblastine [35]. Hepatic metabolism and bile excretion play major roles in the elimination of both vinblastine and vincristine in humans [36]; small quantities of vincristine and vinblastine, in the order of 10% of the administered dose, are excreted with no alterations through urine. The renal clearance of vinblastine is reported as being less than 10% of the total elimination of the serum [37]. It has been reported that vinblastine inhibits a polymorphic cytochrome P-450 in human hepatic microsomes, but the necessary concentrations were higher than those observed in clinical adjustments [38]. It is recommended that vinblastine and vincristine doses must be reduced in patients with liver disease. Vincristine is conventionally administered intravenously, in adults, with a dose of 1.4 mg/m^2, the total dose must not exceed 2 mg in each administration. Sulkes and Collins have commented on the adjustments that can be provided for conventional doses of vincristine and other drugs [39]. Of particular importance is the possibility that some patients can show a good clinical response and relatively low toxicity in dose regimes involving the cautious use of large quantities of vincristine. The initial dose of vinblastine for adults is 3.7 mg/m^2, with a range of the typical growing dose of 5.5–7.4 mg/m^2, administered weekly [37, 38].

5.2 Antidiabetic activity

Considering the traditional use against diabetes, *C. roseus* was included in a research program in Canada, with the objective of finding insulin substitutes. Nevertheless, although no extract derived from the plant showed sensitivity in that regard, an occasional observation in blood indicated that some leaf-derived extracts accumulated alkaloids, sensibly decreasing the number of white globules, granulocytes in particular. This finding motivated scientists to carry out *in vitro* studies with leukemia cells, which lead to the isolation of vinblastine and vincristine in the 60s, among the more than 70 alkaloids of indolic nature that this plant produces. Later, Svodoba in Lilly successfully performed assays in rats with P-1534 leukemia, finding that the tumor was sensitive to these extracts. *Catharanthus roseus* (L.) G. Don is a plant traditionally used by populations in India, South Africa, China, and Malaysia to treat diabetes. Most of the reports on the antidiabetic activity of this plant have been made using crude extracts [39–42].

Soon et al. [43] found that the dichloromethane leaf extract of *Catharanthus roseus* (L.) G. Don showed antidiabetic activity, with an increase in glucose uptake in pancreas (β-TC6) and myoblastic cells (C$_2$C$_{12}$). Four alkaloids—vindoline I, vindolidine II, vindolicine III and vindolinine IV—were isolated and identified from the dichloromethane leaf extract of this plant. The dichloromethane extract and the compounds I–III were not cytotoxic in the pancreatic β-TC6 cells under the highest dose (25.0 µg/mL). The four alkaloids induced a relatively high glucose uptake in pancreatic β-TC6 cells or myoblast C$_2$C$_{12}$, being III the one that showed the highest activity [43, 46, 66].

5.3 Antileukemic activity

Vincristine is employed to treat lymphocytic acute leukemia (the most frequent malign hemopathy in childhood), of which several chromosomic alterations with prognostic importance are known. Among them there are the translocation (4;11) and the translocation (9;22), which are indicators of a bad prognosis, while hyperdiploidy is associated with a good prognosis [44] and it attacks lymphomas including solid tumors in children.

5.4 Antioxidant enzymatic activity

An experiment with different concentrations of sodium chloride in two varieties of *Catharanthus* (var. *alba* and *rosea*) was carried out. It was found that the enzymatic activity of the superoxide dismutase increased at levels of 50 mM of sodium chloride, which helps to raise the levels of this enzyme with antioxidant value [45].

5.5 Antiviral activity

Ozcelik et al. [46] showed the antiviral effect of *Catharanthus* in the simplex herpes virus (type I) with a cytopathogenicity effect at 0.8 μg/mL. Catharoseumine, a monoterpenoid indole alkaloid, has a unique peroxy bridge, which was identified as a potential inhibitor against falcipain-2 protozoa parasites (causes of malaria), showing an IC_{50} value of 4.06 μM. Vinblastine and vincristine showed an antiparasitic effect against *Trypanosoma*, that causes trypanosomiasis in humans, inhibiting its mitosis and affecting its cellular shape in a dose-dependent manner. The use of 15 μM of vinblastine and 50 μM of vincristine inhibited cellular division and cytokinesis, and affected cellular morphology, while the effect of 3 μM of vinblastine and 10 μM of vincristine inhibited cytokinesis without affecting cell cycle progression [46].

5.6 Hypoglycemic activity

It was shown in several animal studies, that ethanolic leaf and flowers extracts decreased the levels of glucose in blood. Hypoglycemic effects are a result of increasing the use of glucose in liver [47]. The aqueous extract decreased glucose in blood in approximately 20% of diabetic rats, compared to methane and dichloromethane extracts in which glucose in blood decreased 49–58% [48]. In the present there are new alkaloids that have been studied in the *Catharanthus* plant, for example, vindogentianine, an hypoglycemic metabolite extracted from leaves, showed hypoglycemic activity in β-TC_6 and C_2C_{12} cells by induction of a higher glucose consumption and a significant *in vitro* inhibition, suggesting that the hypoglycemic activity of vindogentianine is due to the increase in glucose consumption and PTP-1B-type inhibition, which can be a potential therapeutical agent against typ. 2 diabetes [49].

5.7 Antidiarrhoeic *in vivo* activity

The antidiarrhoeic *in vivo* activity of ethanolic leaf extracts was tested in Wistar rats with beaver oil as an experimental diarrhea inductor agent. Loperamide and atropine were used as standard drugs. The antidiarrhoeic effect of the ethanolic extract showed a dose-dependent inhibition of the beaver oil, inducing diarrhea at doses of 200 and 500 mg/kg [50].

5.8 Antimicrobial activity

The antimicrobial activity of leaf extracts was tested against microorganisms such as *Pseudomonas*, *Salmonella*, *Staphylococcus* and thus, these extracts show promissory effects as prophylactic agents in the treatment of many diseases. Ramya et al. [53] evaluated the *in vitro* antibacterial activity through the use of crude extracts of *Catharanthus* [51].

The results indicated that leaf extracts showed a higher antibacterial activity than the extracts prepared from other parts of the *Catharanthus* plant. Thus, the aqueous extracts of leaves, stems, roots and flowers showed low microorganism growth [52] tested leaf extracts of *Catharanthus* var. *rosea*, which showed an excellent activity against *Aspergillus*. Stem extracts of var. *alba* showed a maximum inhibitory activity against *Bacillus* while the flowers of *Catharanthus* var. *rosea* showed a higher activity against *Bacillus* in the methanolic extract. The MIC (Minimal Inhibitory Concentration) against the tested microorganisms was in the range of 100–20 mg/mL. In a different study, foliar acetonic, ethanolic, and chloroformic extracts were tested against pathogenic microorganisms to determine its antimicrobial potential. The ethanolic extract showed the maximum antibacterial activity when compared to the acetonic and chloroformic extracts, in such a way that *Staphylococcus* was the most susceptible bacteria, followed by *Escherichia*, *Pseudomonas* and *Streptococcus* [53].

5.9 Antineoplastic effect

Catharanthus plants contain a series of dimeric indole alkaloids with significant antitumor activities. It has been found that these alkaloids have an *in vitro* and *in vivo* apoptosis-inductive activity against tumor cells, mediated by the nuclear factor kappa potentiator of B activated cells, and by the c-Jun N-terminal kinase pathways, in which DNA damage and mitochondrial dysfunction play important roles. The nuclear factor kappa B was discovered approximately 20 years ago, as a protein that binds to the enhancer of the κ light chain of immunoglobulins in B cells. It belongs to the family of NF-κB transcription factors, which is ubiquitous and participates in the immune and inflammatory response, during tumor development, formation, progression, and apoptosis [54]. The c-Jun N-terminal kinases, originally identified as kinases that bind to and phosphorylate c-Jun protein in the Ser63 and Ser73 residues in their transcriptional activation domain are mitogen-activated kinases responding to stress stimuli, such as cytokinases, UV radiation, thermal shock, and osmotic shock, and are involved both in T lymphocyte differentiation processes, and in apoptosis processes. Different percentages of the crude methanolic extracts have been found to show significant anticancer activity against several cell types under *in vitro* conditions and with a high activity against multidrug-resistant tumor types. On the other hand, Ruskin and Aruna showed that the ethanolic extract of *Catharanthus* has *in vivo* antitumor activity in the Ehrlich carcinoma tumor model, while the *in vitro* study of the ethanolic extract showed significant antitumor activity [55].

6. Extraction and analysis of alkaloids of *Catharanthus roseus*

The extraction method of terpenoid indole alkaloids in *C. roseus* has been optimized by different authors. Most of the methods are time-consuming extractions with several steps and a high use of organic solvents. Despite the high aggregated value of the product, these multi-step processes generate a great amount of organic and acid residues, and as a consequence they rise production cost [56].

Some effective alkaloid extraction methods have been identified from pilose roots of *C. roseus*. For example, Tikhomiroff and Jolicoeur use methanol, lyophilize, dry the roots, and extract during 1 h in a sonication bath [57] use methanol, lyophilize, mash the roots, extract with 45 mL for 5 h in a sonication bath, and evaporate the mobile phase, use methanol and ethyl acetate, extract methanol during 20 min in a sonication bath at 50°C, evaporate methanol, resuspend with 20 mL 0.1 N of HCl, extract with 20 mL of ethyl acetate, adjust pH to 10, evaporate and resuspend in methanol extract with methanol and lyophilize [58]. Extraction can be made from dry material in water with sulfuric acid and four purification stages: fractioning by partition with benzene, two chromatographic columns and finally, crystallization in ethanol and sulfuric acid. Vinblastine and vincristine have been isolated in pure form to be detected through the use of several chromatographic techniques such as: Vacuum Liquid Chromatography with a silica gel column; aluminum oxide (1:1) mixed with Vacuum Liquid Chromatography (VLC); carbon column and purification by accelerated radial chromatography by centrifugation (chromatotron). Semi-quantitative methods have been established by the use of Thin Layer Chromatography (TLC) methods. TLC has a higher sensitivity for alkaloid detection; ajmalicine is detected at a 0.0007% in a volume of 10 μL. Vincristine is detected at 0.055% in a volume of 10 μL, while vinblastine and vindoline are not sensitive to this method since they are both in concentrations of 0.05% in a volume of 10 μL. The chromogenic reactive that is chromatographically used in alkaloid detection is the Cerium Ammonium Sulfate (CAS), which is known for reacting with analyte to produce visible colors in the TLC plate [59].

7. Generalities of the *in vitro* culture

The general process of the *in vitro* culture consists in inoculation on a gelified culture media (generally with agar Gelrite or Phytagel®) with a fragment of plant tissue or an organ, called explant, previously treated to eliminate all the organisms found in its surface (disinfestation). The culture is incubated under controlled environmental conditions of light, temperature, and humidity, that together with the physiochemical and nutritional conditions lead to the development of the explant towards the formation of an amorphous cell mass called callus, or towards the differentiation in an organized tissue that will produce organs or embryos. Organ cultures can be re-differentiated into complete plants (micropropagation) that can be later transferred to a greenhouse, a phase known as acclimation. Culture temperature generally is controlled between 25 and 28°C, the pH between 5.2 and 6.5, and the light from 0 to 12,000 lux. Several studies have researched the effects of pH on cell growth and metabolite production in cell suspension cultures [60].

In addition, several studies modify the pH of the culture media to increase the release of secondary metabolites, and few studies have been carried out to examine the effects of buffers in plant culture growth or in secondary metabolism biosynthesis pathways. Several authors have studied the effect of buffers in *in vitro* cultures of *Catharanthus* roots, to quantify the content of serpentine, ajmalicine, tabersonine, lochnericine, and horhammericine. The main alkaloids serpentine, lochnericine, and horhammericine from *C. roseus* are shown in **Figure 2**.

Light is a very important factor in the *in vitro* production of secondary metabolites of *Catharanthus*. In that regard, other authors showed that temperature has an important influence on cell suspension culture growth and ajmalicine production. The optimal temperature for both biomass growth and secondary metabolite

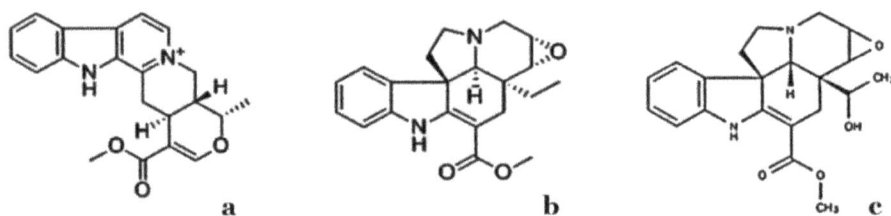

Figure 2.
Alkaloids produced by C. roseus (1) serpentine ($C_{21}H_{21}N_2O_3$, 349.4 g/mol); (2) lochnericine ($C_{21}H_{24}N_2O_3$, 352.43 g/mol) and (3) horhammericine ($C_{21}H_{24}N_2O_4$, 368.42 g/mol).

production is 27.5°C. Young or developing plants with meristematic tissues and vigorous vegetal growth are the best source of explants. Although both juvenile and adult growth can be found in the same plant, the former is characterized by its activity and by the absence of reproductive structures, while the adult growth is slower and presents sexual structures for plant reproduction. The disinfestation of the tissue to be used as a source of explants is made with disinfestant agents like sodium or calcium hypochlorite. The penetration of the disinfestant agent in rugged or hairy surfaces of the plant tissue can increase with the addition of tensioactive agents such as Tween 20. Activated carbon or citric acid are used as antioxidants [61]. In addition, the *in vitro* cultures allow us to know the production of secondary metabolites. In this respect, the sources from which the different *Catharanthus* alkaloids have been isolated *in vitro* are diverse; for example, the alkaloid ajmalicine has been extracted through the analysis from calli, cell suspensions, sprouts, and pilose roots; alstonine from *in vitro* calli; antirhine in cell suspensions; cathindine in suspensions; serpentine in calli, suspensions, sprouts, and pilose roots; acuamicine in calli, suspensions, and sprouts; lochnericine in calli, suspensions, and pilose roots; horhammericine in suspensions and sprouts; tabersonine in calli and suspensions; vindoline in suspensions and sprouts; catharanthine in suspensions, sprouts, and roots; 3,4 anhydrovinblastine in sprouts; catharine in sprouts; vinblastine in calli, sprouts, and somatic embryos; and vincristine in sprouts and embryos, among others [61].

7.1 *In vitro* culture of alkaloid production of *Catharanthus roseus*

It stands out that among the major advantages of plant cell and tissue cultures in basic research, of micropropagation and production of compounds with biologic activity such as secondary metabolites, proteins, and transgenic products, they allow studies in a shorter time and under more controlled conditions than the ones used in traditional methods. A callus is defined as a groups of dedifferentiated friable cells growing in a solid medium and it is the initial material for the estab-lishment and growth of suspension cells. The obtained calli can be subcultured for its maintenance and propagation or induced into differentiation to form organs (organogenesis), embryos (embryogenesis) or to be transferred into a liquid culture medium to obtain cells and small aggregates in suspension. The *in vitro* culture of plant cells in a liquid medium for cell suspensions is a potential source of substance of interest for the pharmaceutical industry, showing all the advantages inherent to biotechnological processes. The advantages offered by cell culture, specifically cell suspension culture, is that it allows a similar handling to the one performed with microorganisms, a fast cell multiplication (duplication time), and it is possible to carry out an scaling into new techniques such as bioreactors and temporal immer-sion systems. However, not all compounds are produced in undifferentiated cells in the same quantity and quality than the ones obtained from mother cells. This is due to many metabolites being synthesized integrally to differentiation events. Several authors have pointed out the identification of cell lines that can produce metabolites in the same amount, or higher, than in natural conditions. New substances have also been detected, which are not synthesized by the plants in their natural environment, which is why it is asserted that cell lines culture constitutes a highly relevant biotechnology for the obtention of new secondary metabolites. *In vitro* cell suspension cultures are kept under the same physical and physicochemical conditions used for calli induction.

There are different *in vitro* culture techniques of the medicinal *C. roseus* plant, which provides a range of important secondary metabolites of pharmacological application, such as the antileukemic alkaloids vinblastine and vincristine, useful in leukemia treatment [62]. Specifically, in cell suspension cultures of *Catharanthus*, all the terpenoid indole alkaloids derivate from an intermediary like strictosidine, including serpentine, catharanthine, ajmalicine, tabersonine, vincristine, and vinblastine [63]. Once the cell culture has been established, a continuous process of epigenetic or genetic changes is observed, which causes the population to be heterogeneous. This creates the necessity of selecting clones with a high growth rate and with a high production of metabolites of interest. Cell lines are obtained through the selection of several strategies, including microscopic (cell viability, for example, with fluorescein diacetate), macroscopic, and enzymatic tests. The aspects associated to secondary metabolites accumulation are the presence of certain cell types, organelles, biosynthetic, or catabolic gene expression and regulation. Thus, organ culture represents an interesting alternative to the production of plant secondary metabolites. Two types of organs are considered to be of greater importance: sprouts and roots, which can be cultivated at a large scale. Organ culture can produce substances of interest that have been obtained through undifferentiated cultures. However, sprout cultures cannot produce all the compounds that are obtained in plant leaves under natural conditions. If the compound of interest is synthesized in roots, then it will not appear in sprouts cultures. On the other hand, it is necessary to take into account that, even though the compound is synthesized in leaves, it is possible that its patterns and concentration are different to the ones obtained from intact plants. As a major advantage, it is pointed out that organ cultures is more genetically stable compared with cell suspension and calli cultures [64].

Several *in vitro* culture techniques such as adventitious meristems or organ propagation, cell and tissue cultures, provide a large amount of *Catharanthus* material for the isolation of mono and dimeric indole type alkaloids with multitherapeutic properties. Several studies have shown that *Catharanthus* is regenerated generally through somatic organogenesis by the induction of friable calli. In addition, *in vitro* cultures of multiple sprouts can be directly induced. Vindoline is an important alkaloid in *in vitro* cultures of *Catharanthus* sprouts. Some authors obtained 2 mg g^{-1} of dry weight after 27 days of culture [65]. Roots synthesize, accumulate, and secrete a large variety of secondary metabolites, in addition to providing mechanical support and allowing water and soil nutrients uptake. It is known that biosynthetic activity in roots is also maintained in *in vitro* cultures. *In vitro* cultures of *Catharanthus* with fast growth have been established in Murashige & Skoog (MS) medium. Several studies mention that *in vitro* cultures are able to synthesize metabolites through root production. These cultures could be a biotechnological alternative of alkaloid production for future research.

Mekky et al. [66] cultured leaves of *C. roseus* in Murashige & Skoog medium supplemented with 1.5 mg/L of BAP and 1.5 mg/L of 2,4-D. The callus obtained was subcultured in 15 different combinations of growth hormones during 28 days.

Alkaloids were extracted from the calli and different treatments were analyzed with HPLC in regard to the capacity of vincristine and vinblastine production compared to the wild plant. Biomass was maximized with combinations of the growth hormone 2,4-D/NAA and IAA/NAA but alkaloid biosynthesis was reduced to the minimum. Vincristine production was potentiated in almost all growth hormone combinations with Kin/IAA, and they produced the highest concentration. However, vinblastine was potentiated in the combinations of growth hormones Kin/IAA, IAA/Gb, BAP/Gb and NAA/Gb only; with Kin/IAA being the one that showed the highest concentration of vinblastine. The main motivating result was the biosynthesis of dimeric anticancer alkaloid essence, vincristine was barely detected in the wild plant and vinblastine, that showed an increase of 3.39-fold compared with the wild plant. In addition, there is a growing demand for these two alkaloids [66].

8. Conclusions

C. roseus is an important medicinal plant with several applications in pharmaceutical and industrial products. In the present, vinblastine and vincristine are two alkaloids for the treatment of childhood leukemia and Hodgkin lymphoma. Production rate of vinblastine and vincristine in *C. roseus* is very low, its extraction costly, and too inefficient to be industrialized. The semisynthesis also faces many obstacles because of the necessary presence of precursors and intermediaries. The great pharmacological importance of the terpenoid indole alkaloids vincristine and vinblastine, associated to its low content in plants (approximately 0.0005% of dry weight), *in vitro* tissue and cell cultures, will permit the stimulation of intense research regarding the biosynthesis pathways of terpenoid indole alkaloids yet unknown through *in vitro* culture studies under biotic or abiotic elicitation strategies with the objective of increasing the production of *C. roseus* alkaloids.

Acknowledgements

This work was supported by the "Programa para el Desarrollo Profesional Docente" PRODEP-Mexico of the project 2017-2018 of Hebert Jair Barrales-Cureño PhD of the Universidad Intercultural del Estado de Puebla.

Conflict of interest

All contributing authors declare no conflict of interest.

List of abbreviations

BAP	6-Benzylaminopurine
CAS	Cerium Ammonium Sulfate
Gb	Gibberellin
HPLC	High-Performance Liquid Chromatography
IAA	Indole-3-acetic acid
KIN	Kinetin
NAA	1-Naphthaleneacetic acid
TIA	Terpenoid indole alkaloids

TLC   Thin Layer Chromatography
VLC   Vacuum Liquid Chromatography
2,4-D   2,4-Dichlorophenoxyacetic acid

Author details

Hebert Jair Barrales-Cureño[1], César Reyes Reyes[1], Irma Vásquez García[1*],
Luis Germán López Valdez[2], Adrián Gómez De Jesús[3], Juan Antonio Cortés Ruíz[4],
Leticia Mónica Sánchez Herrera[5], María Carmina Calderón Caballero[6],
Jesús Antonio Salazar Magallón[7], Jose Espinoza Perez[1] and Jorge Montiel Montoya[8]

1 División de Ciencias Naturales, Ingeniería Forestal Comunitaria, Universidad
Intercultural del Estado de Puebla, Puebla, Mexico

2 Preparatoria Agrícola, Universidad Autónoma Chapingo, Texcoco de Mora,
Mexico

3 CONACYT—Facultad de Ciencias Agronómicas de la Universidad Autónoma de
Chiapas, Villaflores, Chiapas, Mexico

4 Instituto Tecnológico de Mazatlán, Mazatlán, Sinaloa, Mexico

5 Unidad de Tecnología de Alimentos, Universidad Autónoma de Nayarit, Tepic,
Nayarit, Mexico

6 Instituto Tecnológico Superior de Uruapan, Uruapan, Michoacán, Mexico

7 Laboratorio de Control Biológico, Momoxpan, Puebla, Mexico

8 Centro Interdisciplinario de Investigación para el Desarrollo Integral Regional
Unidad Sinaloa, Instituto Politécnico Nacional, Guasave, Sinaloa, Mexico

*Address all correspondence to: irma.vasquez@uiep.edu.mx

IntechOpen

References

[1] Saiman MZ, Miettinen K, Mustafa NR, Choi YH, Verpoorte R. Metabolic alteration of *Catharanthus roseus* cell suspension cultures overexpressing geraniol synthase in the plastids or cytosol. Plant Cell Tissue and Organ Culture. 2018;**134**:41-53. DOI: 10.1007/s11240-018-1398-5

[2] Aslam J, Khan SH, Siddiqui ZH, Zohra F, Maqsood M, Bhat MA, et al. *Catharanthus roseus* (L.) G. Don. An important drug: It's applications and production. Pharmacie Globale. 2010;**1**(4):1-17

[3] Acosta LL, Rodríguez FC. Instructivo técnico para el cultivo de *Catharanthus roseus* (L.) G. Don Vicaria. Revista Cubana de Plantas Medicinales. 2002;**7**: 96-99

[4] Alor CMJ, Gómez AR, Huerta LE, Pat FJM, González CM, De la Cruz GC. Nutrición y crecimiento en fase de vivero de *Catharanthus roseus* (L.) G. Don, *Mimordica charantia* L. y *Azadirachta indica* A. Juss, en el Municipio Centro, Tabasco–México. Boletín Latinoamericano y del Caribe de. Plantas Medicinales y Aromáticas. 2012;**11**:163-171

[5] Schlaepfer L, Mendoza-Espinoza JA. Las plantas medicinales en la lucha contra el cáncer, relevancia para México. Revista Mexicana de Ciencias Farmacéuticas. 2010;**41**:18-27

[6] Gomes de Moraes L, Alonso AM, Oliveira-Filho EC. Plantas medicinais no tratamento do câncer: Uma breve revisão de literatura. Universitas: Ciências da Saúde, Brasília. 2011;**9**: 77-99. DOI: 10.5102/ucs.v9i1.1308

[7] Gobbi GP, Ferreri JMA, Ponzoni M, Levis A. Hodgkin lymphoma. Critical Reviews in Oncology/Hematology. 2013;**85**:216-237. DOI: 10.1016/j. critrevonc.2012.07.002

[8] Warwick OH, Darte JMM, Brown TC. Some biological effects of vincaleukoblastine, an alkaloid in *Vinca rosea* Linn in patients with malignant disease. Cancer Research. 1960;**20**: 1032-1040

[9] Johnson IS, Wrigh HF, Svoboda GH, Vlantis J. Antitumor principles derived from *Vinca rosea* Linn I. Vincaleukoblastine and Leurosine. Cancer Research. 1960;**20**:1017-1022

[10] Neumann B, Hu W, Nigro K, Gilliam AC. Agressive histiocytic disorders that can involve the skin. Journal of the American Academy of Dermatology. 2007;**56**:302-316. DOI: 10.1016/j.jaad.2006.06.010

[11] Smith H, Qualls C, Prairie B, Padilla LA, Rayburn WF, Key CR. Trends in gestational choriocarcinoma: A 27 year perspective. Obstetrics and Gynecology. 2003;**102**:978-987. DOI: 10.1016/S0029-7844(03)00669-0

[12] Rojo EA. Sarcoma de Kaposi: Revisión de la literatura e ilustración de un caso. Acta Médica Grupo Ángeles. 2013;**11**:23-31

[13] Lewis WH. Plants for man: Their potential in human health. Canadian Journal of Botany. 1982;**60**:310-315

[14] Chakraborty T, Poddar G. Herbal drugs in diabetes. Part I: Hypoglycaemic activity of indigenous plants in *Streptozotocin* (Stz.) induced diabetic rats. Journal of the Institution of Chemists. 1984;**56**:20. DOI: 10.1590/S0102-695X2007000200005

[15] Loyola-Vargas VM, Sánchez-Iturbe P, Canto-Canché B, Gutiérrez-Pacheco L, Gálaz-Ávalos R, Moreno-Valenzuela O. Biosíntesis de los alcaloides indólicos. Una revisión crítica. Revista de la Sociedad Química de Mexico. 2004;**48**:67-94

[16] Sottomayor M, Lopes Cardoso I, Pereira LG, Barceló A. Peroxidase and the biosynthesis of terpenoid indole alkaloids in the medicinal plant *Catharanthus roseus* (L.) G. Don. Phytochemistry Reviews. 2004;**3**: 159-171. DOI: 10.1023/B: PHYT.0000047807.66887.09

[17] Levingston R, Zamora R. Medicine trees of the tropic. Unasylva. 1983;**35**: 7-10

[18] Naeem M, Aftab T, Masroor KMA. *Catharanthus roseus*. Current Research and Future Prospects. India: Springer; 2017. 412 p. DOI: 10.1007/978-3-319-51620-2

[19] Fuentes V, Granda M. Conozca Las Plantas Medicinales. La Habana: Ed. Científico-Técnica; 1997. p. 244

[20] Acosta L. Proporciónese salud. In: Cultive Plantas Medicinales. La Habana: Ed. Científico-Técnica; 1995. p. 227

[21] Barrales-Cureño HJ. Aplicaciones farmacológicas y producción biotecnológica in vitro de los alcaloides anticancerígenos de Catharanthus roseus. Biotecnologia Aplicada. 2015;**32**: 1101-1110

[22] Starobova H, Vetter I. Pathophysiology of chemotherapy-induced peripheral neuropathy. Frontiers in Molecular Neuroscience. 2017;**31**(10):174. DOI: 10.3389/fnmol.2017.00174

[23] Van der Fits L, Memelink J. ORCA3, a jasmonate-responsive transcriptional regulator of plant primary and secondary metabolism. Science. 2000; **289**:295-297. DOI: 10.1126/science.289.5477.295

[24] De Luca V. Enzymology of indole alkaloid biosynthesis. Methods in Plant Biochemistry. 1993;**9**:345-368. DOI: 10.1007/978-1-4757-0097-84

[25] Goddijn OJM, Pennings EJM, Van der Helm P, Schilperoort RA, Verpoorte R, Hoge JHC. Overexpression of a tryptophan decarboxylase cDNA in *Catharanthus roseus* crown gall cultures results in increased tryptamine leveis but not in increased terpenoid indole alkaloid production. Transgenic Research. 1995;**4**:315-323. DOI: 10.1007/BF01972528

[26] Zhu J, Wang M, Wen W, Yu R. Biosynthesis and regulation of terpenoid indole alkaloids in *Catharanthus roseus*. Pharmacognosy Reviews. 2015;**9**:24-28. DOI: 10.4103/0973-7847.156323

[27] De Luca V, Fernandez JA, Campbell D, Kurz WGW. Developmental regulation of enzymes of indole alkaloid biosynthesis in *Catharanthus roseus*. Plant Physiology. 1988;**86**:447-450. DOI: 10.1104/pp.86.2.447

[28] Liscombe DK, OConnor SE. A virus-induced gene silencing approach to understanding alkaloid metabolism in *Catharanthus roseus*. Phytochemistry. 2011;**72**:1969-1977. DOI: 10.1016/j.phytochem.2011.07.001

[29] Verpoorte R, Van der Heijden R, Ten Hopeen HJG, Memelink J. Metabolic engineering of plant secondary metabolic pathways for the production of fine chemicals. Biotechnology Letters. 1999;**21**:467-479. DOI: 10.1023/A:1005502632053

[30] St-Pierre B, Vázquez-Flota FA, De Luca V. Multicellular compartmentation of *Catharanthus roseus* alkaloid biosynthesis predicts intercellular translocation of a pathway intermediate. Plant Cell. 1999;**11**:887-900. DOI: 10.1105/tpc.11.5.887

[31] Ouwerkerk PBF, Memelink J. Elicitor responsive promoter regions in the tryptophan decarboxylase gene from *Catharanthus roseus*. Plant Molecular Biology. 1999b;**39**:129-136. DOI: 10.1023/A:1006138601744

[32] Menke FLH, Parchmann S, Mueller MJ, Kijne JW, Memelink J. Involvement of the octade-canoic pathway and protein phosphorylation in fungal elicitor-induced expression of terpenoid indole alkaloid biosynthetic genes in *Catharanthus roseus*. Plant Physiology. 1999;**119**:1289-1296

[33] Menke FLH, Champion A, Kijne JW, Memelink J. A novel jasmonate- and elicitor-responsive element in the periwinkle secondary metabolite biosynthetic gene *strl* interacts with a jasmonate and elicitor-inducible AP2-domain transcription factor, ORCA2. The EMBO Journal. 1999;**18**:4455-4463. DOI: 10.1093/emboj/18.16.4455

[34] Vázquez-Flota FA, De Luca V. Jasmonate modulates development- and light-regulated alkaloid biosynthesis in *Catharanthus roseus*. Phytochemistry. 1998;**49**:395-402. DOI: 10.1016/S0031-9422(98)00176-9

[35] Nelson RL, Dyke RW, Root MA. Comparative pharmacokinetics of vindesine, vincristine and vinblastine in patients with cancer. Cancer Treatment Reviews. 1980;7:17-24. DOI: 10.1016/S0305-7372(80)80003-X

[36] Owellen RJ, Hartke CA. The pharmacokinetics of 4-acetyl. Tritium vinblastine in two patients. Cancer Research. 1975;**35**:975-980

[37] Ackland SP, Ratain MJ, Vogelzang NJ, Choi KE, Ruane M, Sinkule JA. Pharmacokinetics and pharmacodynamics of long-term continuous-infusion doxorubicin. Clinical Pharmacology and Therapeutics. 1989;**45**:340-347. DOI: 10.1038/clpt.1989.39

[38] Relling MV, Evabs WE, Fonne-Pfister R, Meyer UA. Anticancer drugs as inhibitors of two polymorphic cytochrome P-450 enzymes, debrisoquine and mephenytoin hydroxylase in human liver microsomes. Cancer Research. 1989;**49**:68-71

[39] Sulkes A, Collins JM. Reappraisal of some dosage adjustment guidelines. Cancer treatment reports. 1987;**71**:229

[40] Ohadoma SC, Michael HU. Effects of co-administration of methanol leaf extract of *Catharanthus roseus* on the hypoglycemic activity of metformin and glibenclamide in rats. Asian Pacific Journal of Tropical Medicine. 2011;**4**: 475-477. DOI: 10.1016/S1995-7645(11)60129-6

[41] Gacche RN, Dhole NA. Profile of aldose reductase inhibition, anti-cataract and free radical scavenging activity of selected medicinal plants: An attempt to standardize the botanicals for amelioration of diabetes complications. Food and Chemical Toxicology. 2011;**49**:1806-1813. DOI: 10.1016/j.fct.2011.04.032

[42] Ganga RM, Satyanarayana S, Eswar KK. Safety of Gliclazide with the aqueous extract of *Vinca rosea* on pharmacodynamic activity in normal and alloxan induced diabetic rats. Journal of Pharmacy Research. 2012;**5**: 1555-1558

[43] Soon HT, Chung YL, Hazrina H, Aditya A, Mohammadjavad P, Won FW, et al. Antidiabetic and antioxidant properties of alkaloids from *Catharanthus roseus* (L.) G Don. Molecules. 2013;**18**:9770-9784. DOI: 10.3390/molecules18089770

[44] Rubnitz JE, Behm FG, Pui CH, Evans WE, Relling MV, Raimondi SC, et al. Genetic studies of childhood acute lymphoblastic leukemia with emphasis on p16, MLL and ETV6 gene abnormalities: Results of St Jude total therapy study XII. Leukemia. 1997;**11**: 1201-1206

[45] Abdul JC. Soil salinity regimes alters antioxidant enzyme activities in two

varieties of *Catharanthus roseus*. Botany Research International. 2009;**2**:64-68

[46] Ozcelik B, Kartal M, Orhan I. Cytotoxicity, antiviral and antimicrobial activities of alkaloids, flavonoids, and phenolics acids. Pharmaceutical Biology. 2011;**49**:396-402. DOI: 10.3109/13880209.2010.519390

[47] Chattopadhyay RR. A comparative evaluation of some blood sugar lowering agents of plant origin. Journal of Ethnopharmacology. 1991;**67**:367-372. DOI: 10.1016/S0378-8741(99)00095-1

[48] Singh SN, Vats P, Suri S. Effect of an antidiabetic extract of *Catharanthus roseus* on enzymic activities in streptozotocin induced diabetic rats. Journal of Ethnopharmacology. 2001;**76**:269-277. DOI: 10.1016/S0378-8741(01)00254-9

[49] Tiong SH, Looi CY, Arya A, Wong WF, Hazni H, Mustafa MR, et al. Vindogentianine, a hypoglycemic alkaloid from *Catharanthus roseus* (L.) G. Don (Apocynaceae). Fitoterapia. 2015;**102**:182-188. DOI: 10.1016/j.supflu.2017.03.018 10.5897/AJPP11.505

[50] Kyakulaga A, Hassan AT, Brenda VP. *In vivo* antidiarrheal activity of the ethanolic leaf extract of *Catharanthus roseus* Linn. (Apocynaceae) in Wistar rats. African Journal of Pharmacy and Pharmacology. 2011;**5**:1797-1800. DOI: 10.1016/j.supflu.2017.03.018 10.5897/AJPP11.505

[51] Naz S, Haq R, Aslam F, IIyas S. Evaluation of antimicrobial activity of extracts of *in vivo* and *in vitro* grown *Vinca rosea* L. (*Catharanthus roseus*) against pathogens. Pakistan Journal of Pharmaceutical Sciences. 2015;**28**:849-853

[52] Kumari K, Gupta S. Antifungal properties of leaf extract of *Catharanthus roseus* L (g.) Don. American Journal of Phytomedicine and Clinical Therapeutics. 2013;**1**:698-705

[53] Ramya S, Govindaraji V, Navaneetha KK, Jayakumararaj R. *In vitro* evaluation of antibacterial activity using crude extracts of *Catharanthus roseus* L. (G.) Don. Ethnobotanical Leaflets. 2008;**12**:1067-1072

[54] Echeverri RNP, Mockus SI. Factor nuclear κB (NF-κB): Signalosoma y su importancia en enfermedades inflamatorias y cáncer. Revista de la Facultad de Medicina. 2008;**56**:133-146

[55] Ruskin RS, Aruna SR. *In-vitro* and *in-vivo* antitumor activity of *Catharanthus roseus*. International Research Journal of Pharmaceutical and Applied Sciences. 2014;**4**:1-4

[56] Falcao MA, Scopel R, Almeida RN, do Espirito SAT, Franceschini G, Garcez JJ, et al. Supercritical fluid extraction of vinblastine from *Catharanthus roseus*. The Journal of Supercritical Fluids. 2017;**129**:9-15. DOI: 10.1016/j.supflu.2017.03.018

[57] Tikhomiroff C, Jolicoeur M. Screening of *Catharanthus roseus* secondary metabolites by high-performance liquid chromatography. Journal of Chromatography. 2002;**955**:87-93. DOI: 10.1016/S0021-9673(02)00204-2

[58] Bhadra R, Vani S, Shanks JV. Production of indole alkaloids by selected hairy root lines of *Catharanthus roseus*. Biotechnology and Bioengineering. 1993;**41**:581-592. DOI: 10.1002/bit.260410511

[59] Magagula NL, Mohanlall V, Odhav B. Optimized thin layer chromatographic method for screening pharmaceutically valuable alkaloids of *Catharanthus roseus* (Madagascar Periwinkle). International Journal of Sciences. 2012;**12**:1-20

[60] Morgan J, Barney C, Penn A, Shanks J. Effects of buffered media

upon growth and alkaloid production of *Catharanthus roseus* hairy roots. Applied Microbiology and Biotechnology. 2000; **53**:262-265. DOI: 10.1007/s002530050018

[61] Van der Heijden R, Jacobs DI, Snocijer W, Hallard D, Verpoorte R. The *Catharanthus alkaloids*: Pharmacognosy and biotechnology. Current Medicinal Chemistry. 2004;**11**:607-628. DOI: 10.2174/0929867043455846

[62] Shams KA, Nazif NM, Abdel ASA, Abdel SKA, El-Missiry MM, Ismail SI, et al. Isolation and characterization of antineoplasic alkaloids from *Catharanthus roseus* L. Don. cultivated in Egypt. African Journal of Traditional, Complementary, and Alternative Medicines. 2009;**6**:118-122

[63] El-Sayed M, Verpoorte R. *Catharanthus* terpenoid indole alkaloids: Biosynthesis and regulation. Phytochemistry Reviews. 2007;**6**: 277-305. DOI: 10.1007/s11101-006-9047-8

[64] Bourgaud F, Gravot A, Milesi S, Gontier E. Production of plant secondary metabolites: A historical perspective. Plant Science. 2001;**161**: 839-851. DOI: 10.1016/S0168-9452(01)00490-3

[65] Hernández-Domínguez E, Campos-Tamayo F, Vázquez-Flota F. Vindoline synthesis in *in vitro* shoot cultures of *Catharanthus roseus*. Biotechnology Letters. 2004;**26**:671-674. DOI: 10.1023/B:BILE.0000023028.21985.07

[66] Mekky H, Al-Sabahi J, Abdel-Kreem MFM. Potentiating biosynthesis of the anticancer alkaloids vincristine and vinblastine in callus cultures of *Catharanthus roseus*. South African Journal of Botany. 2018;**114**:29-31. DOI: 10.1016/j.sajb.2017.10.008

Chapter 3

Synthesis of Tropane Derivatives

Abdulmajeed Salih Hamad Alsamarrai

Abstract

This chapter refers to tropane alkaloid compounds best known for their occurrence, biosynthesis, and pharmacological properties in a subsection of the plant
family Solanaceae including the *Atropa*, *Duboisia*, *Hyoscyamus*, and *Scopolia* species,
together with their semisynthetic derivatives. Tropane alkaloids are useful as
parasympatholytics that competitively antagonize acetylcholine. The bicyclic ring
of tropane moiety forms the base of these alkaloids, and the largest number of
tropane alkaloids is substituted on the atom C-3 of the tropane ring in the form
of ester derivatives. Also, this chapter provides routes to previous methods for
synthesizing tropane-2-yl derivatives as well as new routes to synthesize
2-(*p*-toluenesulphonyl) tropane-2-ene (anhydroecgonine). The new strategy for
synthesizing anhydroecgonine might be helpful to adopt the best method of
synthesizing tropane-2-yl derivatives.

Keywords: alkaloids, tropane, ecgonine, cocaine, tropinone, tropidine

1. Introduction

1.1 Tropane alkaloids occurrence

Tropane alkaloids (**Figure 1**) are among the oldest medicines known to men.
A secondary metabolites containing the tropane nucleus constitute one of the
largest and most important group of naturally occurring compounds [1]. Secondary
metabolites of Solanaceae plant, sharing tropane skeleton (1) as a common structural feature can be divided into two classes: tropine (2) and ecgonine (3) derivatives [2]. The first group is represented by atropine from *Atropa belladonna* (4) and
scopolamine (5) (*Scopola carniolica*) which are considered to be anticholinergic
drugs. The second includes one of the strong stimulants and mostly used as a
recreational drug, cocaine (6).

Over 600 naturally occurring alkaloids of tropane can be found in plants such as
Datura stramonium [3]. Cocaine (6) was first isolated from *Erythroxylon coca* in
1860 [4–7] and is still a prolific field of research. Although alkaloids with the
tropane moiety are the oldest medicines known to man, they are still a subject
of continual review in the chemical literature, and only recently they have been
isolated, purified, and studied [8, 9].

1.2 Biosynthesis of tropane alkaloids

Alkaloids possess quite complex structures, and the study of biosynthesis of
these alkaloids has a long history. It is generally thought that the tropane moiety
arises from complex enzymatic processes involving phytochemical precursors.

(1) Tropane

(2) Tropine

(3) Ecgonine

(4) Atropine

(5) Scopolamine

(6) Cocaine

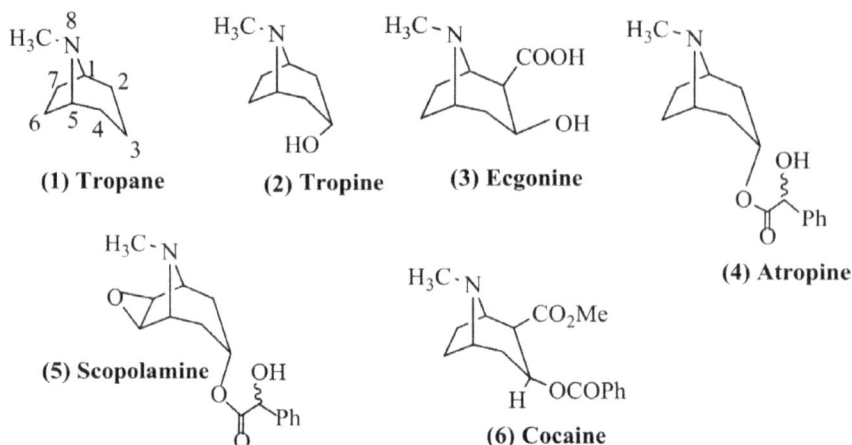

Figure 1.
Some tropane alkaloids.

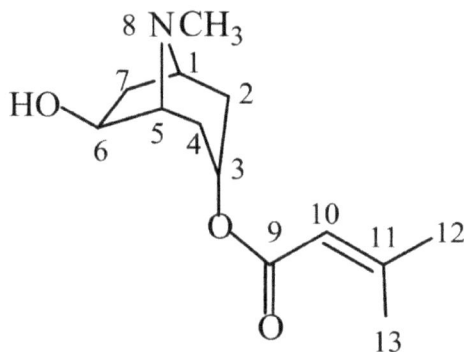

8 NCH₃

Figure 2.
3 Alpha-senecioyloxy-6beta-hydroxytropane.

Incorporation of radioactive labeled precursors has eased monitoring pathway on which the tropane derivatives are formed [10]. Recent studies making use of labeled ornithine (7), N-methylornithine (8), and 1,4-butanediamine (9) prepared biosynthetically, have firmly established these precursors and representative examples of complex tropane alkaloids found in Solanaceae plant [11]. After the establishment of the origins of these precursors, attention has been directed mainly toward those alkaloids which, in addition to the tropane residue, contain a 9- or 10-carbon atom unit such as 3α-senecioyloxy-6β-tropane (see **Figure 2**). These units exist in many variant forms, but certain recurrent features led to the belief that many variants have a common phytochemical precursors, for instance, L-ornithine (7) is believed to be converted to diamine (9) by specific enzyme such as hyoscyamine-6β-hydroxylase (H6H) and the former (9) is considered the precursor in biosynthesis of the bicyclic [3.2.1] skeleton of tropane alkaloids which is outlined in **Figure 3**.

It has been found that oxidation of tropane ring can be achieved by molecular oxygen in the presence of ferrous ions. Also, it has been found that these keto forms of tropane can be catalyzed by an enzyme called reductase [12]. For instance, the biosynthesis pathway to tropane alkaloids, tropinone (10), is reduced by reductase to tropine (2), as it can be seen in **Figure 4**.

Structural assignments of tropane molecules have exhibited difficult problems, and, as a result, progress in their endeavors has been closely associated with

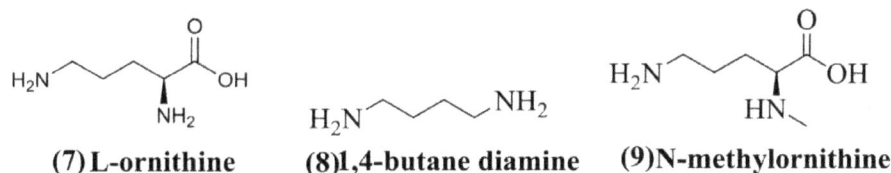

(7) L-ornithine   **(8)1,4-butane diamine**   **(9)N-methylornithine**

Figure 3.
Amino acids precursors in the biosynthesis of tropane skeeton.

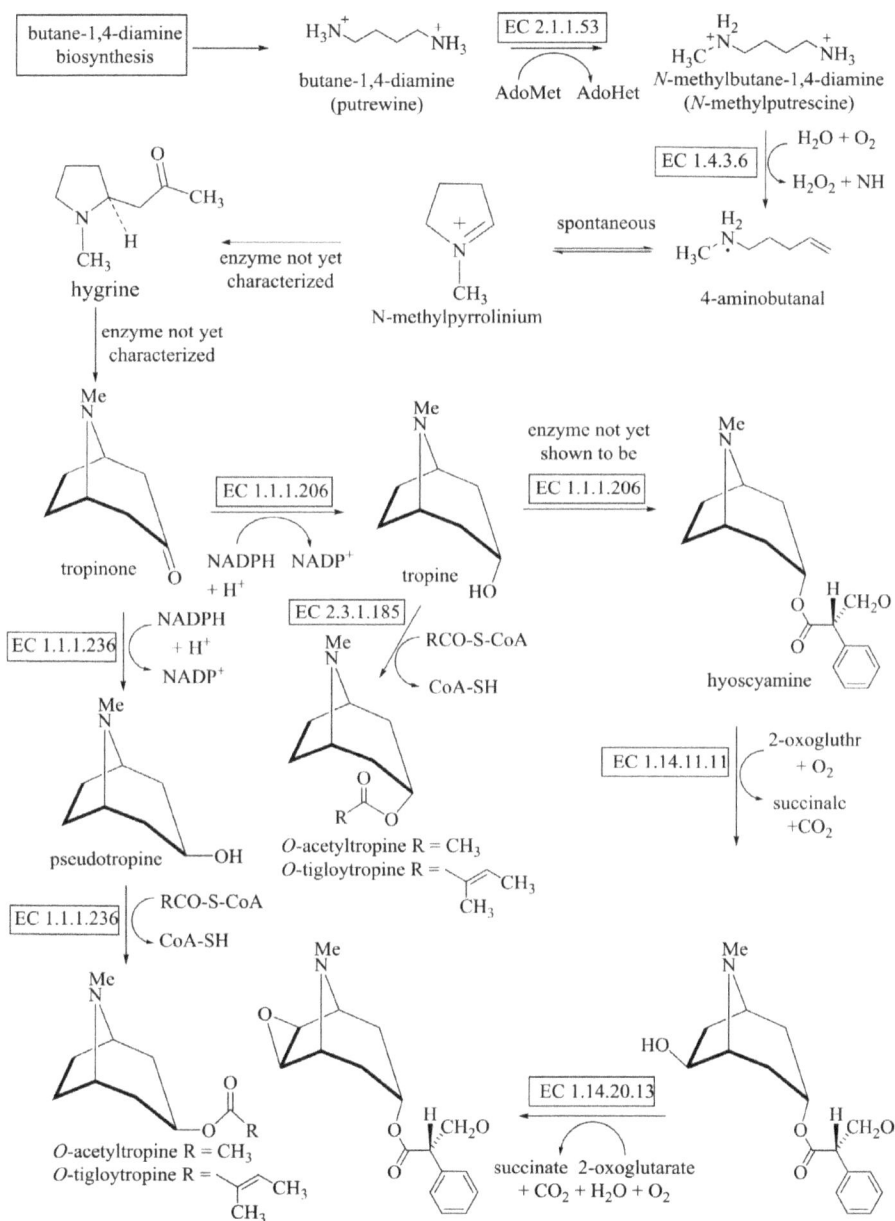

Figure 4.
Bio-synthesis of tropane alkaloids-Alcheetron.com-760 × 570.

development of modern analytical techniques of spectroscopy, of which mass spectroscopy deserves particular mention such as ESI MS, GC-MS, HPLC-MS, and MALDI MS.

1.3 Pharmacological properties of tropane alkaloids

Concerning the pharmacological effects, these compounds are so important because of their pharmacological properties [13]. Alkaloids such as atropine (4), scopolamine (5), and cocaine (6) and their derivatives are best recognized to have pharmacological actions related in the body to the function of neurotransmitter acetylcholine [14]. Some tropane alkaloids can act as anticholinergic effects or stimulants [15]. Pharmaceuticals of tropane derivatives are economically important. Over 20 active pharmaceutical ingredients containing tropane moiety in their structures are manufactured and used as antispasmodics, anesthetic, and mydriatics (see **Figure 5**) [16].

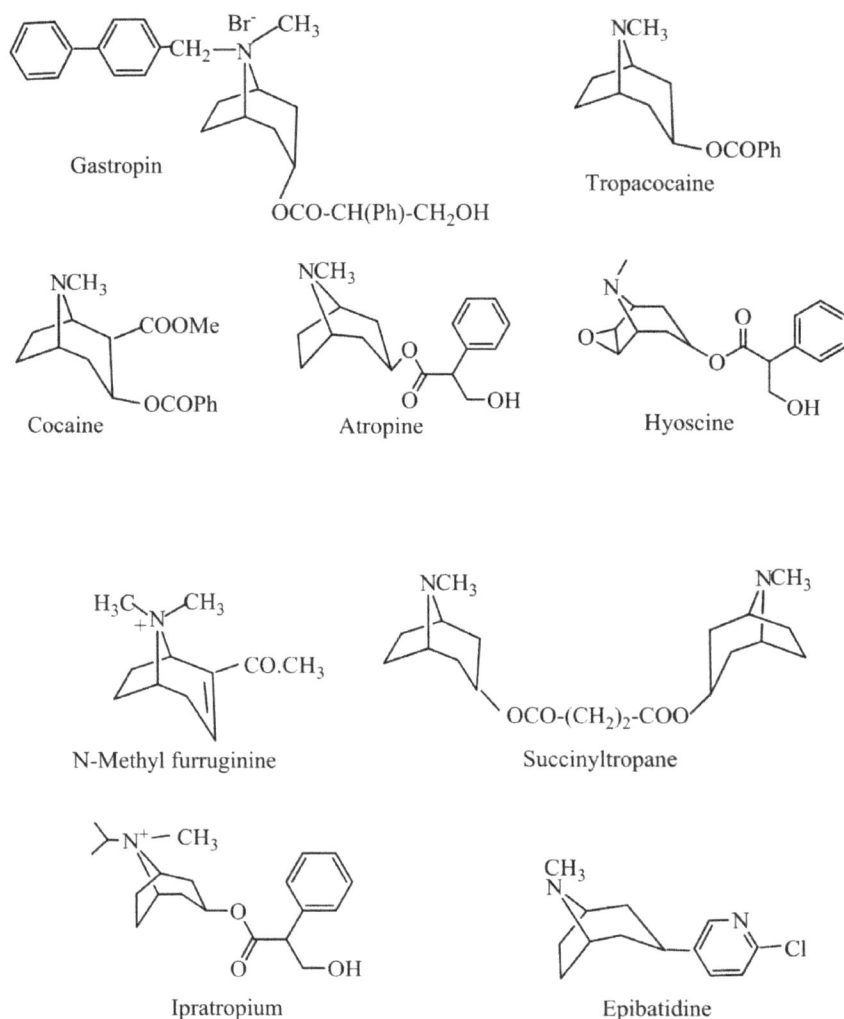

Figure 5.
Some pharmaceutical ingredients containing tropane moiety.

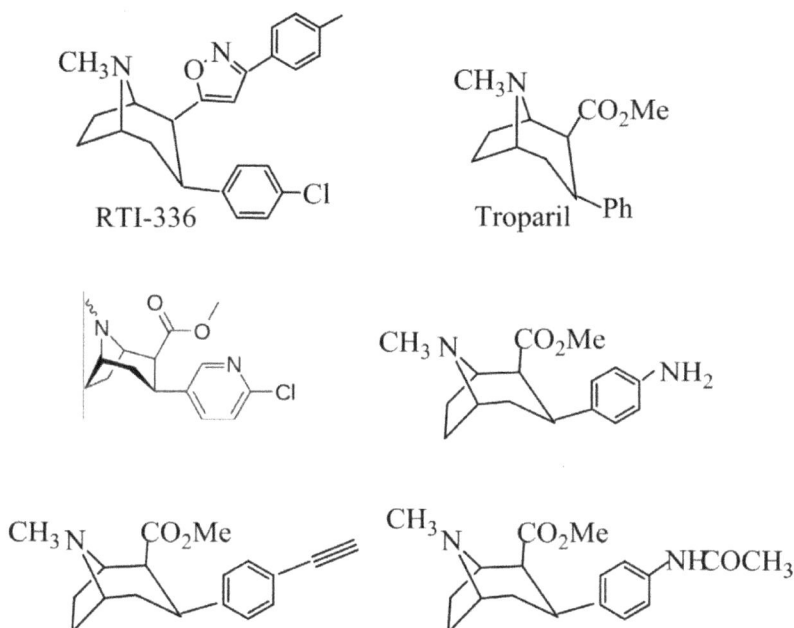

Figure 6.
Some phenyl tropane compounds.

Tropane does not occur naturally in free forms. The favored forms of tropane in plant species are the esters forms. These esters are generally secondary metabolites of the plant species. Tropane esters were isolated from different plant families like Proteaceae, Rhizophoraceae, Euphorbiaceae, and Convolvulaceae, and they are well known to occur in Solanaceae. Most tropane alkaloids in the Solanaceae family arises from the esterification of acids, such as acetic acid, propanoic acid, isobutyric acid, isovaleric acid, 2-methylbutyric acid, tifilic acid (+)-α-hydroxyl-β-phenylpropionic acid, tropic acid, and atropic acid with various hydroxytropanes (α-tropane-diol or α-tropane-triol) [5]. Almost all of the tropane-based pharmaceuticals are natural or semisynthetic esters [5, 17, 18]. There are also alkylated or arylated tropane compounds known as phenyltropane (**Figure 6**).

2. Chemistry of tropane alkaloid synthesis routes

Although there are many synthetic routes, Robinsons one-pot synthesis of tropane and its derivatives designed in 1917 [19] is still the best choice for the synthesis of such compounds. The parameters have been changed from time to time in order to increase yield to synthesize a specific derivative (**Figure 7**).

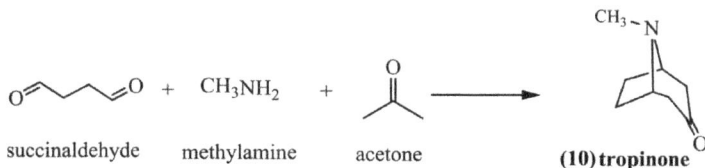

Figure 7.
Robinson's one pot synthesis of tropinone (10).

2.1 Synthesis of tropan-2-yl derivatives

The naturally occurring alkaloid, cocaine (6), possesses a functional group at C-2 in the tropane ring system, which has been modified to give various 2-aminotropanes. Willstatter [20], in his work devoted to the elucidation of the structure of ecgonine (3), obtained the amide (11) which it degraded by Hofmann reaction to 2α-aminotropane (12) (the α-configurations retained throughout this sequence can be assigned for later work) (**Figure 8**) [21].

Willstatter also obtained (12) by Curtius reaction of the ester (13), and this reaction has been used earlier by Fodor [22] to obtain the amino alcohols (14) and (15), although, again, the configurations at C-2 and C-3 were not known when the work was carried out (**Figure 9**).

Apart from these isolated examples, the most consistent interest in 2-substituted tropanes was shown in connection with the alkaloid dioscorine (16), which was for some time thought to have structure (17) and therefore to be related to tropan-2-one (18). This ketone is an optically active form, which was first prepared by Bell and Archer from ecgonine (3) (**Figure 10**) [23].

The action of phosphoryl chloride on ecgonine (3) was shown by Einborn to give the acid chloride of anhydroecgonine (19) [24]. Bell and Archer converted the crude acid chloride directly to the corresponding amide (20), from which L-(+)-tropan-2-one (18) was obtained in fair yield by Hofmann reaction (**Figure 11**).

When this material was compared with the ketone obtained by degradation of dioscorine (16), the two could not be distinguished [25], and it was left to Pinder and his co-workers to prove that dioscorine was not in fact a tropane derivative [26]. Pinder found that tropidine (21) reacts with the more usual peracid oxidizing

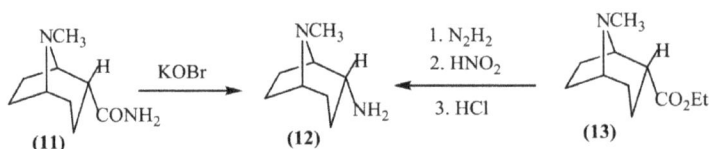

Figure 8.
Hoffmann of the amide (11) to the (12).

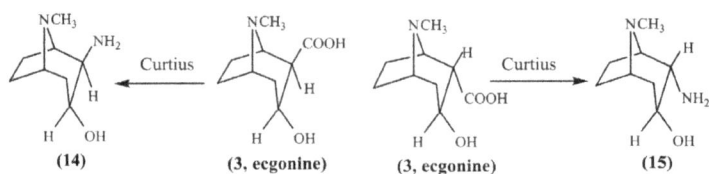

Figure 9.
Curtius reduction of ecgonine to amino alcohols (14) and (15).

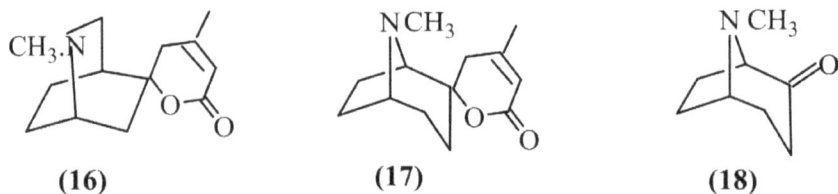

Figure 10.
Some 2-substituted tropane alkaloids.

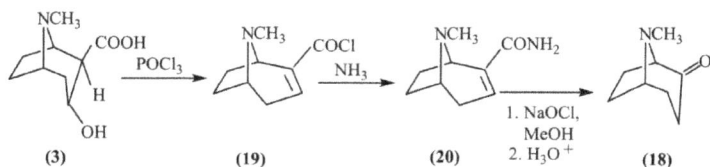

Figure 11.
Synthesis of tropane-2-one.

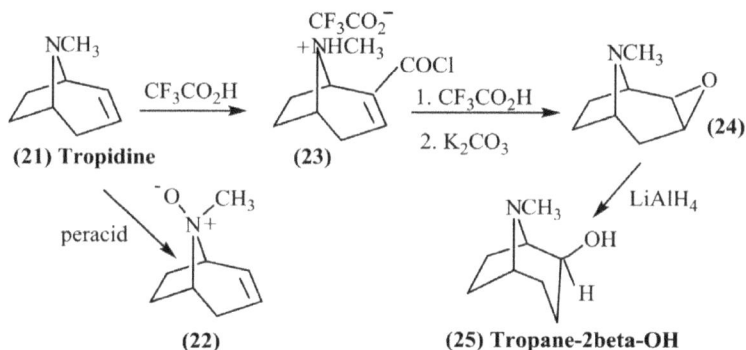

Figure 12.
Synthesis of tropane-beta-ol (25).

agents to give the N-oxide (22), and in acid solution no reaction took place [27]. However, the action of trifluoroperacetic acid on tropidine trifluoroacetate salt (23) gave the 2β,3β-epoxide (24). Reduction of the epoxide with lithium aluminum hydride yielded tropan-3-β-o1 (25), but it was found impossible to oxidize this amino alcohol to tropan-2-one (18) (Figure 12).

A synthesis of the desired ketone was eventually achieved by a larger route. Treatment of 2-ethoxycarbonyl-pyrrole (26) with phosphoryl chloride and dimethylformide yielded the two isomeric aldehydes, (27) and (28), which were separated fairly easily by fractional distillation in vacuum. Thereafter the crucial stage, a Dieckmann cyclization, led to the β-ketoester (29), which hydrolyzed and was decarboxylated to tropan-2-one (18), outlined in Figure 13 [26].

Pinder resolved the racemic product into its optically active components and discovered that (+)-tropan-2-one (18) was quite different from the ketone derived from the alkaloid dioscorine (16). With this demonstration that dioscorine (16) was not a tropane derivative, the interest in 2-substituted tropanes diminished, and few papers concerned with these compounds have appeared since 1962.

Tropane-2-one (18) is a convenient source of both tropan-2-αβ-ols. Reduction of the ketone with lithium aluminum hydride yields tropan-2α-ol (25), which is the expected, equatorial product [23, 26]. Reduction of a cyclic ketone with sodium alcohol mixtures also usually gives the thermodynamically more stable, equatorial alcohol [28], but with sodium in propan-2-ol, pentan-3-ol, tropan-2-one gave mixtures of tropan-2β-ol (30) and tropan-2α-ol (25) [23] (Figures 13 and 14). Moreover, when the ratio of alcohol to alkoxide ion at the end of the reaction was increased, the product was found to contain increasing amounts up to 90% of tropan-2β-ol (30). These facts suggested that the axial alcohol (25) is more stable thermodynamically, and this was confirmed by subjecting the pure equatorial isomer (25) to equilibration by means of sodium 2-pentoxide in pentan-3-ol containing 10% fluorenone: the equilibrium mixture contained 85% of the axial isomer (25) [23].

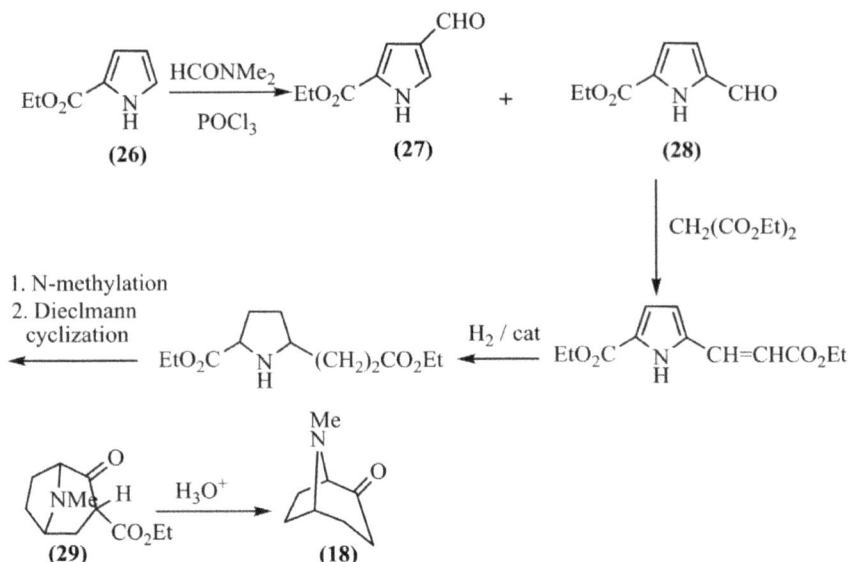

Figure 13.
Synthesis of tropane-2-one (18).

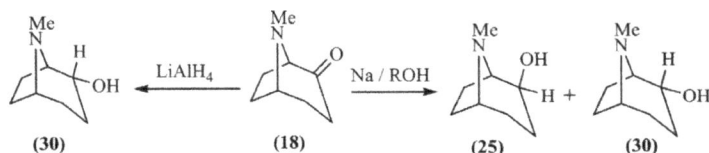

Figure 14.
Synthesis of tropane-2-ol (30).

This reversal of the usual axial equatorial stability relationship may be attributed to the presence of strong, intramolecular hydrogen bonding between the axial hydroxyl group and the nitrogen bridge (31). When the possibility of hydrogen bond formation is removed, as in the anions (32) and (33), the equatorial configuration becomes more stable. When the ratio of free alcohol to alkoxide ion at the end of the sodium alcohol reduction is large, the equilibrium will be mainly between the two alcohols (25) and (30); in these conditions, the product will contain a high proportion of the more stable, axial alcohol. Conversely, when the final proportion of alkoxide ion in the reaction mixture is high, a significant equilibrium between anions (32) and (33) will exist, and the product will contain a higher proportion of the equatorial alcohol (30), arising from the more stable anion (32) (**Figure 15**). These stability relationships enable a useful control of the product ratio to be exercised.

Two further preparations, of 2-halotropanes, are worthy of note. Nickon found that the addition of 1 molar equivalent of bromine to a methanolic solution of tropinone (10) yielded a granular complex, which rearranged to 2β-bromotropinone (34), by spontaneous transition under ether or by acid catalysis [29]. Earlier, Hobson and Riddell obtained 2β-chlorotropane (36) by decomposition of the *N*-chloramine (35) in the presence of silver ion (**Figure 16**) [30, 31]. The identical chlorotropane was also obtained by chlorination of the mine hydrochloride, followed by cyclization of the dichloride (37).

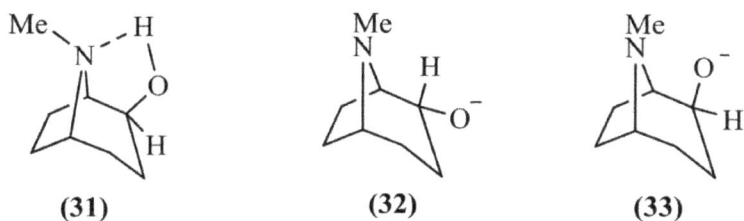

Figure 15.
The stability relationship of the products (25) and (30).

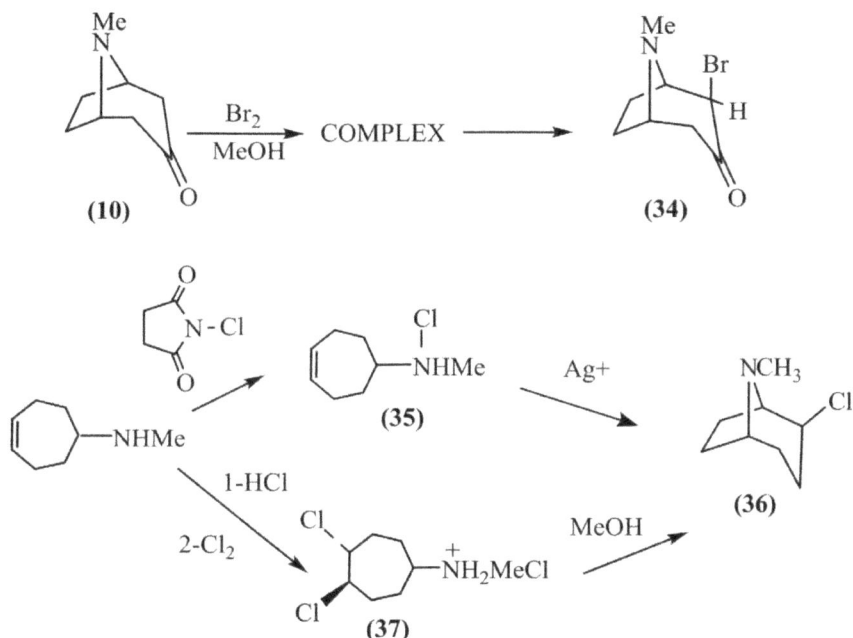

Figure 16.
Synthesis of 2-bromo-3-tropinone (34) and the 2-chlorotropane (36).

Although tropan-2-one (18) appeared to be a very convenient synthetic precursor of both tropan-2α-ol (30) and tropan-2β-ol (25), the ketone itself was not easy to prepare. The ketone may be obtained in good yield from ecgonine (3) or cocaine (6), but these alkaloids are expensive. The alternative starting material used by Pinder and co-workers, 2-ethoxycarbonyl-pyrrole (26), is also expensive, and the subsequent synthesis was too long for it to be useful for the preparation of large amount of tropan-2-one.

2.2 Synthesis of tropan-2β-ol (21) from tropinone (10)

Tropinone (10) was available in reasonable quantities and was chosen as a convenient source of tropane derivatives. Reduction of this ketone with borohydride gave a mixture of the epimeric tropan-3-ols (38), which were dehydrated to tropidine (21) by Landenburg's method [31] as it can be seen in **Figure 17**.

An allylic oxidation of tropidine (21) with selenium dioxide [32] to yield a β-unsaturated ketone (39) was an attractive prospect, but this could not be realized: there was no apparent reaction in aqueous dioxin after 50 hours on a boiling water bath. Other allylic reagents, such as N-bromosuccinimide or lead tetraacetate,

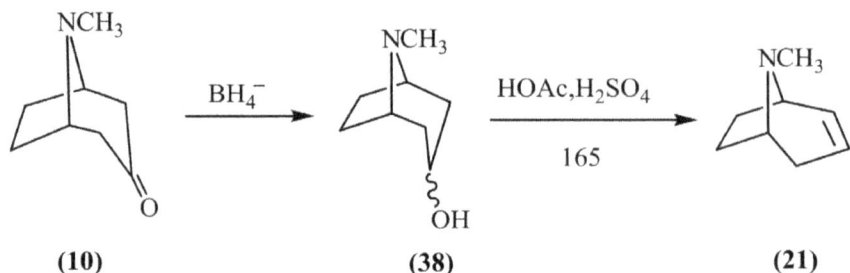

Figure 17.
Synthesis of tropidine (21) from Tropane-3-one.

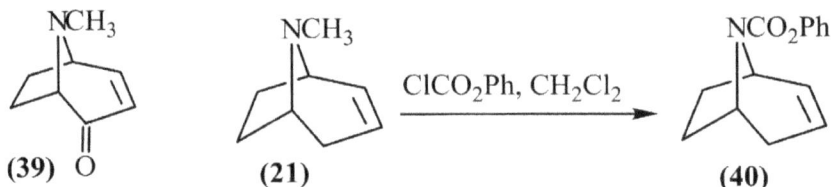

Figure 18.
Synthesis of the compound (40).

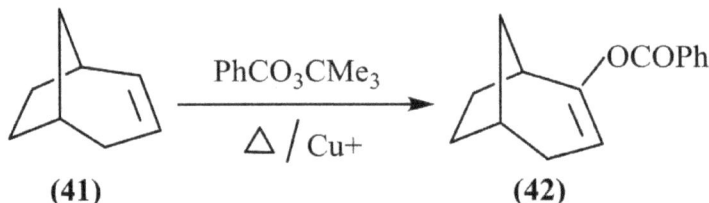

Figure 19.
Synthesis of the racemic mixture of (42).

would also be ineffectual in the presence of the N-methyl group, so that the most convenient method of protecting the nitrogen atom is provided by the reaction of tropane derivative with phenyl chloroformate [33]; thus, treatment of tropidine (21) with phenyl chloroformate in dichloromethane gave N-phenoxycarbonyl-nor-tropidine (40) a good yield (**Figure 18**). The nitrogen of the urethane group is non-basic, and, furthermore, the N-methyl group can be regenerated by reduction of the urethane with lithium aluminum hydride.

Goering and Mayer [34] have reported that optically pure bicyclo[3.2.1]oct-2-ene (41) reacts with tert-butyl perbenzoate, in the presence of cuprous ion, to give racemic of (42) presumably via a symmetrical allyl radical (**Figure 19**).

Epoxidation of unreactive olefins with trifluoroperacetic acid is usually carried out in dichloromethane with phosphate present to buffer the trifluoroacetic acid that is a product of the reaction [35]. The epoxidation of N-phenoxycarbonyl-nor-tropidine (40) by means of trifluoroperacetic acid was inconvenient for two reasons. Firstly, it gave a mixture of products, including a large proportion of unchanged olefin, which necessitated careful column chromatography of the mixture in order to obtain the required 2β,3β-epoxide (43a, b) (**Figure 20**). Secondly, the peracid itself is inconvenient to prepare and is an unpleasant reagent. It has been reported that there is a simplified procedure for epoxidation, using a nitrile as a

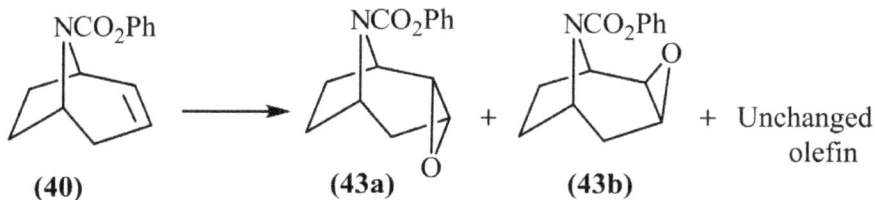

Figure 20.
Synthesis of the epoxides of (40).

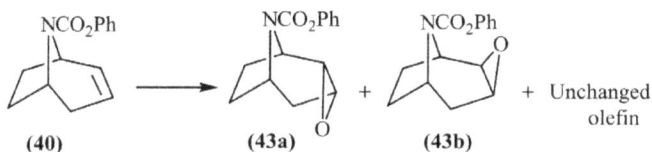

Scheme (13): synthesis of the epoxides of (40)

$$RCN + H_2O_2 \xrightarrow[\text{OH}^-]{\text{pH 8}} RC(=NH)OOH$$

$$RC(=NH)OOH + Reagent \longrightarrow RC(O)NH_2 + \text{Oxidation product}$$

$$RC(=NH)OOH + H_2O_2 \longrightarrow R\text{-}C(O)\text{-}NH_2 + O_2 + H_2O$$

Figure 21.
Synthesis of peroxycarboximidic acid.

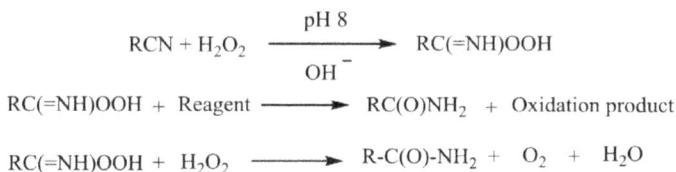

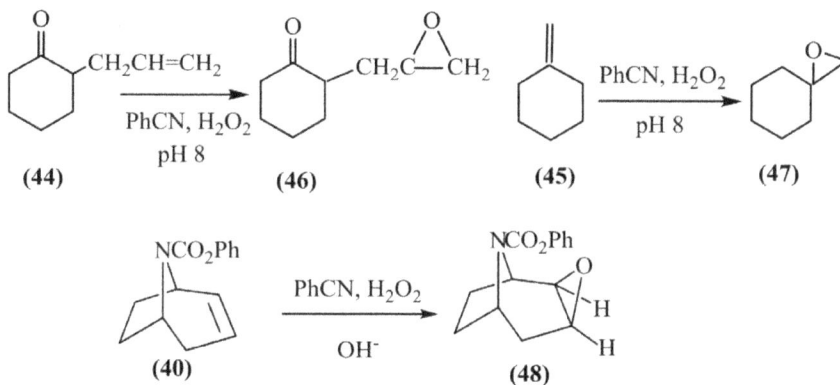

Figure 22.
Oxidation of some unreactive olefines.

reactant with hydrogen peroxide [36, 37]. The reaction occurs in weekly basic solution and is thought to involve a peroxycarboximidic acid [RC(=NH)OOH], which is too reactive to be isolated. In the absence of a suitable reducing agent, [RC(=NH)OOH] will oxidize hydrogen peroxide, the Radziszewski reaction [38] outlined in **Figure 21**. But in the presence of an olefin, the Radziszewski reaction may be eliminated and epoxidation effected [36].

For example, the epoxidations of (44) and (45) proceeded smoothly with benzonitrile and hydrogen peroxide to (46) and (47), respectively (**Figure 22**), whereas (44) was found to undergo Baeyer-Villiger cleavage with peracetic acid [41]. The reaction of *N*-phenoxycarbonyl-nor-tropidine (40) with benzonitrile and hydrogen peroxide in weakly basic solution gave the expected 2β,3β-epoxide (48). By the use of a large excess of reagents, a yield of 38% was achieved but could not be increased [39].

2.3 Synthesis of 2-(*p*-toluenesulphonyl) tropane-2-ene: anhydroecgonine analog

As mentioned earlier, molecules that contained tropane structure, for example, tropane (1), ecgonine (2), tropinone (3), and cocaine (4) or one of its fragments, show central stimulating effects [40–45], using them as anticholinergic agents [46, 47].

Much of the modification designs involved isomeric studies [48]. Most of the modifications came to the tropane moiety, the bridge nitrogen (N_8) [49], or modification at the C_2 position [50]. Many processes for synthesizing anhydroecgonine derivatives without using cocaine as a starting material have been reported in literature. For example, it was shown by Grundmann and Ottman [51] as well as Okano and Osamu [52] that the reaction of ethyl cycloheptatriene-7-carboxylate (49) with methylamine gave anhydroecgonine ethyl ester (50) (**Figure 23**). Conversion of the corresponding carboxylic acid to tropane-2-one has been accomplished by Bell and Archer [53] in a four-step sequence involving conversion to the carboxamide and Hofmann degradation with sodium hypochlorite.

Because (49) was not readily available, Hobson et al. [54] as well as Okano and Itoh [55] developed a relatively inexpensive route starting with corresponding cyano-derivatives which is readily accessible by reaction of tropylium fluoroborate (51) with sodium cyanide to give (52). The nitrile (52) was reacted with methylamine in t-butanol to give the 2-cyano tropidine (53) in high yield (see **Figure 24**).

In our work on the 1,3,5-cycloheptatriene-2-ylphosphorus derivatives (54) and (55) (**Figure 25**), little success was achieved in obtaining isolable products from reactions with nitrogen nucleophiles, except in those cases, for example, pyrrole2-aldehyde, where the presence of aldehyde group enabled the intermediate ylide to be trapped [56].

Investigation of the behavior of the 2-(*p*-toluenesulphonyl) analog in this type of reaction turned out to be more fruitful and provided a useful entry to 2-substituted tropanes, and in particular the rather difficultly accessible ketone, tropan-2-one. 7-(*p*-Toluenesulphonyl)-1,3,5-cycloheptatriene (56) was found to react smoothly with primary amines in dry acetonitrile under reflux to give adducts of general structure (57) in good yields, thus greatly improving the accessibility of compounds of this type [57]. When (56) was isomerized to (56a) in acetnitrile using 1,4-diazabicyclo[2.2.2] octane (DABCO) as a catalyst, and the latter was treated with methylamine in refluxing ethanolic solution, 2-(*p*-toluenesulphonyl)-8-methyl-8-azabicyclo[3.2.1] oct-2-ene (57a) was obtained as a pale yellow oil in a yield of 80% (**Figure 26**).

Its mass spectrum showed a molecular ion peak at m/e 277, and the IR spectrum showed a band at 1600 cm^{-1} characterizing the double bond. Identification of this compound was confirmed by the ^{1}H-NMR spectrum, which showed signals at δ 3.15

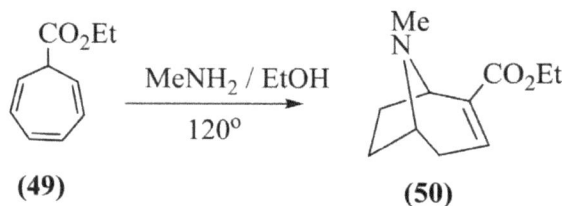

Figure 23.
Synthesis of anhydroecgonine ethyl ester (50).

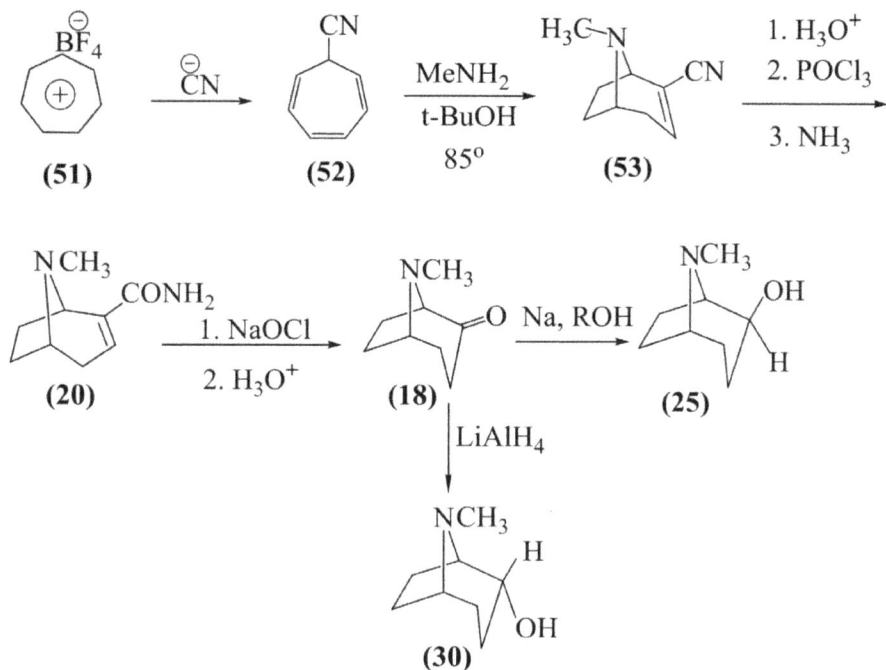

Figure 24.
Synthesis of the acetonitrile (52) and it's conversion to (18).

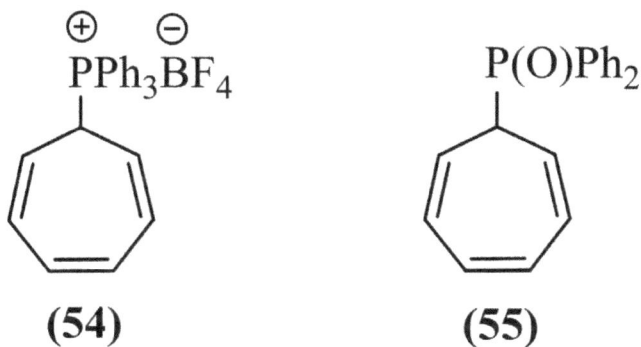

Figure 25.
7-phosphonium and phosphine oxide of cycloheptatriene.

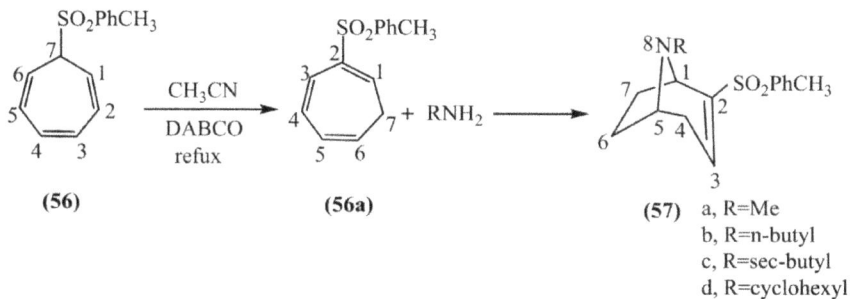

Figure 26.
Synthesis of 2-(p-toluenesulphonyl)-8-methyl-8-azabicyclo[3.2.1]oct-2-ene (57a).

and 3.45 due to the bridgehead protons, H_1 and H_5; a 1-H multiplet at 6.82 as well as upfield protons between 1.2 and 2.8 ppm (see Structure 57, a = Me).

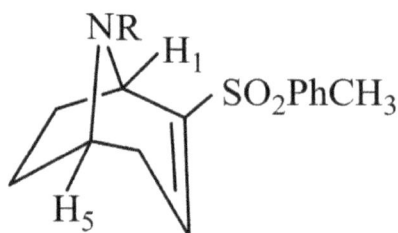

(57, a=Me)

Similarly the sulfone (56a) was refluxed with an excess of *n*-butylamine in acetonitrile; TLC examination showed the formation of only one product. Isolation and recrystallization from hexane afforded white crystals of 2-(*p*-toluenesulphonyl)-8-*n*-butyl-8-azabicyclo[3.2.1]oct-2-ene (57b), mp, 119–121°C (85%.). Mass (m/z 319) and IR and NMR spectra confirmed that the compound was (57b). Another example of this reaction involving addition of sec-butylamine to the sulfone (56b) also proved successful under similar conditions. 2-(*p*-tolylsulphonyl)-8-sec-butyl-8-azabicyclo[3.2.1]oct-2-ene (57c) was obtained in 41% yield as a colorless oil which partially crystalized on standing. TLC analysis of this product showed two inseparable spots for the diastereoisomers of (58) and (59) (**Figure 27**). The NMR spectral data included a multiplet at δ 0.6–2.20 as expected for upfield protons of (57c) accompanied by signals at 3.35, 3.60, and 6.85 ppm due to two bridgehead protons and one olefinic proton, respectively. The elemental analysis and mass spectrum (molecular ion at m/z 319) confirmed the structure. Also, the reaction of the sulfone (56a) with excess of cyclohexylamine in refluxing acetonitrile also gave a solid product in 75% yield 2-(*p*-toluenesulphonyl)-8-cyclohexyl-8-azabicyclo[3.2.1]oct-2-ene (57d). Its IR and NMR spectra were similar with those structures of (57a–c), and the structure was confirmed by the mass spectrum, which showed a molecular ion peak at m/z 345.

In the case of the reaction of (56a) with benzylamine, a slightly different result was obtained. The product was obtained as needles, mp 172°C, and elemental analysis, mass spectroscopy, and spectral data confirmed the structure (60) (**Figure 28**).

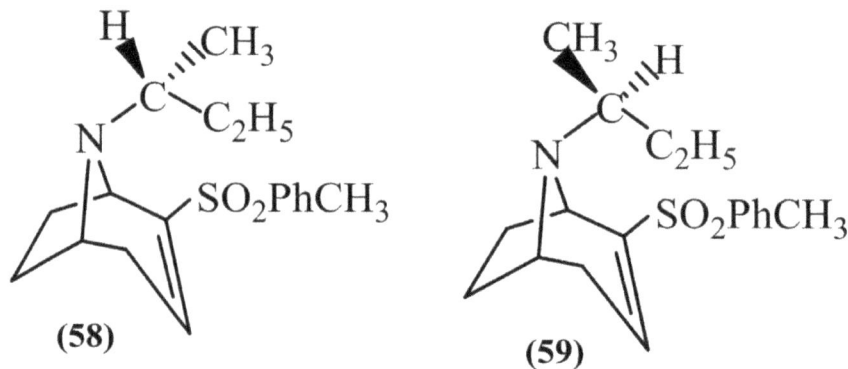

(58)

(59)

Figure 27.
The diastereomers (58) and (59).

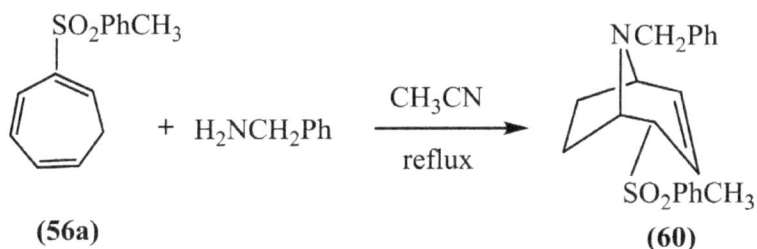

Figure 28.
Synthesis of compound (60).

The mechanism for the formation of compounds (57a–d) and (60) presumably involves in the first step of the Michael addition of the amine to C_1 of the sulfone (56a) to give intermediate compound (61). Further base-catalyzed isomerization gives the compound (62), followed by intramolecular Michael addition which would lead to the compounds (63a–d) and (60) (**Figure 29**). In the case of the compound (63a–d), further isomerization to the conjugated sulfone took place which was presumably facilitated by the presence of the strong bases, methylamine (pKa 10.659), n-butylamine (pKa 10.77), s-butylamine (pKa 10.83), and cyclohexylamine (pKa 10.66). The formation of the kinetically controlled product (60) in the case of the benzylamine reaction was presumably due to the weaker basicity of benzylamine (pKa 9.35) which does not promote further isomerization. The same product was also obtained using acetonitrile as a solvent for the reaction. Cycloheptatriene was also obtained in the reaction mixture, presumably formed by slow decomposition of the sulfone (56a).

The total absence of 2-(p-toluenesulphonyl)-8-t-butyl-8-azabicyclo[3.2.1]oct-2-ene (65) in the products indicated that there was no nucleophilic attack on C_1 of the sulfone (56a) presumably because of steric bulk of the t-butyl substituent (**Figure 30**).

Attempts to react the sulfone (56a) with ammonia were unsuccessful; a solution of the sulfone (58a) in dry acetonitrile was refluxed and ammonia bubbled through for 24 hours. The only product to be isolated was a small quantity of what appeared to be, from its spectral properties, a pure toluene-p-sulphonamide.

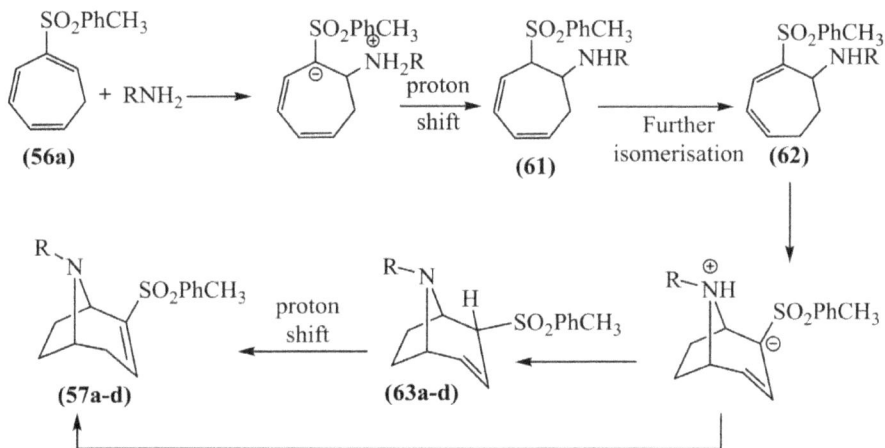

Figure 29.
Synthesis of 2-(p-toluenesulphonyl)-8-azabicyclo[3.2.1]oct-2-ene (57a–d).

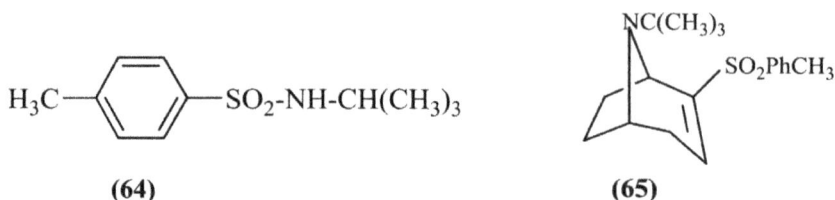

Figure 30.
Show the formation of compound (64) and absence of compound (65).

3. Conclusions

The tropane alkaloids made a great contribution to the history of medicine. Intensive research on chemistry and pharmacology of tropane alkaloids led to a fast development of pharmaceutical industries, particularly drugs that have anticholinergic effects. Since the first one-pot synthesis of tropane-3-one by Robinsons in 1917, several routes for synthesizing semisynthetic and synthetic tropane derivatives were published in literature. Chemical synthetic routes from different disciplines and field of research combined in this chapter, in an attempt to illustrate how through continual research, facilitate and develop synthetic chemistry of tropane derivatives. However, the synthesis of the famous tropane derivative, anhydroecgonine from 7-(p-toluenesulfonyl)-1,3,5-cycloheptatriene and amines, would provide alternative chemical procedure to people working in this field. This procedure has been shown to be simple, inexpensive research, and provide inspiration in the search for more tropane derivatives.

Author details

Abdulmajeed Salih Hamad Alsamarrai
Chemistry Department, College of Applied Sciences, University of Samarra, Samarra, Iraq

*Address all correspondence to: abdulmajeedsalihhamad@yahoo.com

IntechOpen

References

[1] Lounasmaa M, Tamminen T. The tropane alkaloids. In: Cordell GA, editor. The Alkaloids. Vol 44, Chemistry and Pharmacology. New York: Academic Press; 1993. pp. 1-115

[2] Jirschitzka J, Schmidt GW, Bernd MR, Schneider JG, D'Auria JC. Plant tropane alkaloid biosynthesis evolved independently in the Solanaceae and Erythroxylaceae. Proceedings of the National Academy of Sciences of the United States of America. 2012;**109**(26): 10304-10309. DOI: 10.1073/pnas.1200473109

[3] Robins RJ, Abraham TW, Parr AJ, Eagles J, Walton NJ. The biosynthesis of tropane alkaloids in *Datura stramonium*: The identity of the intermediates between *N*-methylpyrrolinium salt and tropinone. Journal of the American Chemical Society. 1997;**119**(45): 10929-10934. DOI: 10.1021/ja964461p

[4] Fodor G. The tropane alkaloids. In: Manske RHF, editor. The Alkaloids; Chemistry and Physiology. Vol. XIII. New York: Academic Press; 1971. pp. 351-396

[5] Gyermek L. Structure-activity relationships among derivatives of dicarboxylic acid esters of tropine. Pharmacology & Therapeutics. 2002; **96**:1-21

[6] Leake CD, Pelikan EW. An historical account of pharmacology to the 20th century (book review). Journal of Clinical Pharmacology. 1976;**16**:669-671

[7] Sneader W. Plant products analogues and compounds derived from them. In: Sneader W, editor. Drug Discovery; A History. Chichester: Wiley & Sons, Ltd; 2005. pp. 115-150

[8] Holmes HL, Manske RHF. The Alkaloids. New York: Academic Press; 1961

[9] Saxton JE. The Alkaloids. New York: Academic Press; 1965

[10] Kitamura Y, AtsukoTaura YK, Miura H. Conversion of phenylalanine and tropic acid into tropane alkaloids by *Duboisia leichhardtii* root cultures. Journal of Plant Physiology. 1992; **140**(2):141-146. DOI: 10.1016/S0176-1617(11)80924-7

[11] Humphrey AJ, O'Hagan D. Tropane alkaloid biosynthesis. A century old problem unresolved. Natural Product Reports. 2001;**18**(5):494-502. DOI: 10.1039/B001713M

[12] Nakaima K, Hashimoto T. Two tropine reductases, that catalyze opposite stereospecific reductions in tropane alkaloid biosynthesis, are localized in plant root with different cell-specific patterns. Plant & Cell Physiology. 1999;**40**:1099-1107

[13] Robins RJ, Walton NJ. The alkaloids: Chemistry and pharmacology. 1993;**44**: 115-187

[14] Camps P, Munoz-Torrero D. Cholinergic drugs in pharmacotherapy of Alzheimer's disease. Mini Reviews in Medicinal Chemistry. 2002;**2**:11-25

[15] Chin YW, Kinghorn AD, Patil PN. Evaluation of the cholinergic and adrenergic effects of two tropane alkaloids from *Erythroxylum pervillei*. Phytotherapy Research. 2007;**21**:1002-1005

[16] Christen P. Tropane alkaloids: Old drugs used in modern medicine. In: Rahman A, editor. Studies in Natural Products Chemistry, Bioactive Natural Products, Part C. Vol. 22. Amsterdam: Elsevier Science and Technology; 2000. pp. 717-749

[17] Majewski M, Lazny R. Synthesis of tropane alkaloids via enantioselective

deprotonation of tropinone. The Journal of Organic Chemistry. 1995;**60**:5825-5830

[18] Maksay G, Nemes P, Biro T. Synthesis of tropeines and allosteric modulation of ionotropic glycine receptors. Journal of Medicinal Chemistry. 2004;**47**:6384-6391

[19] Oksman-Caldentey KM. Tropane and nicotine alkaloid biosynthesis—Novel approach towards biotechnological production of plant derived pharmaceuticals. Current Pharmaceutical Biotechnology. 2007;**8**: 2003-2010

[20] Robinson R. Journal of the Chemical Society, Transactions. 1917;**111**:762-768. DOI: 10.1039/CT9171100762

[21] Willstätter R, Müller W. Ueber die Constitution des Ecgonins. Berichte der Deutschen Chemischen Gesellschaft. 1898;**31**(3):2655-2669

[22] de Jong AWK. Some properties of the ecgonines and their esters. III: The α. β-position of the double bond in ecgonidine, the structural formulae and autoracemisation of the ecgonines. Recueil des Travaux Chimiques des Pays-Bas. 1937;**56**(7):678-680

[23] Fodor G, Kovács Ö. 478. The stereochemistry of the tropane alkaloids. Part III. The configuration of scopolamine and of valeroidine. Journal of the Chemical Society (Resumed). 1953:2341-2344

[24] Bell MR, Archer S. Ethyl 3α-phenyltropane-3β-carboxylate and related compounds. Journal of the American Chemical Society. 1960; **82**(17):4638-4641

[25] Einhorn A. Ueber Ecgonin. Berichte der Deutschen Chemischen Gesellschaft. 1887;**20**(1):1221-1229

[26] Ayer DE, Büchi G, Warnhoff PR, White DM. The structure of dioscorine.

Journal of the American Chemical Society. 1958;**80**(22):6146

[27] Davies WAM, Pinder AR, Morris IG. The synthesis and resolution of (±)-tropan-2-one. Tetrahedron. 1962;**18**(4): 405-412

[28] Davies WAM, Jones JB, Pinder AR. 703. An alkaloid of *Dioscorea hispida*, dennstedt. Part VI. Some investigations on the synthesis of tropan-2-one. Journal of the Chemical Society (Resumed). 1960:3504-3512

[29] Barton DHR. The stereochemistry of cyclohexane derivatives. Journal of the Chemical Society (Resumed). 1953: 1027-1040

[30] Riddell WD. Ph.D. thesis. Birmingham; 1968

[31] Hobson JD, Riddell WD. Transannular cyclisations of cyclo-olefinic N-chloro-amines. Chemical Communications (London). 1968;**19**: 1178-1180

[32] Archer WL, Cavallito CJ, Gray AP. Bisammonium salts. Unsymmetrical derivatives of tropane and related bases1. Journal of the American Chemical Society. 1956;**78**(6):1227-1228

[33] Rabjohn N. Selenium dioxide oxidation. Organic Reactions. 1949;**5**: 331-386

[34] Hobson JD, McCluskey JG. Cleavage of tertiary bases with phenyl chloroformate: The reconversion of 21-deoxyajmaline into ajmaline. Journal of the Chemical Society C: Organic. 1967:2015-2017

[35] Georing HL, Mayer U. Journal of the American Chemical Society. 1964;**88**: 3753-3760

[36] Emmons WD, Pagano AS. Peroxytrifluoroacetic acid. IV. The epoxidation of olefins1. Journal of the

American Chemical Society. 1955;77(1): 89-92

[37] Payne GB, Deming PH, Williams PH. Reactions of hydrogen peroxide. VII. Alkali-catalyzed epoxidation and oxidation using a nitrile as co-reactant. The Journal of Organic Chemistry. 1961; 26(3):659-663

[38] Payne GB. A simplified procedure for epoxidation by benzonitrile-hydrogen peroxide. Selective oxidation of 2-allylcyclohexanone. Tetrahedron. 1962;18(6):763-765

[39] Wiberg KB. The mechanisms of hydrogen peroxide reactions. I. The conversion of benzonitrile to benzamide. Journal of the American Chemical Society. 1953;75(16): 3961-3964

[40] Ogata Y, Sawaki Y. The alkali phosphate-catalyzed epoxidation and oxidation by a mixture of nitrile and hydrogen peroxide. Tetrahedron. 1964; 20(9):2065-2068

[41] Iewin AH, Naseree T, Carroll FI. A practical synthesis of (+) cocaine. Journal of Heterocyclic Chemistry. 1987;24:19-21. DOI: 10.1002/jhet.5570240104

[42] Katoh T, Kakiya K, Nakai T, Nakamura S, Nishide K, Node M. A new divergent synthesis of (+) and (-) ferrugine utilizing PLE-catalysed asymmetric dealkoxycarbonylation. Tetrahedron: Asymmetry. 2002;13: 2351-2358

[43] Lazny R, Sienkiewicz M, Olenski T, Urbanczyk-Lipkowska Z, Kalicki P. Approches to the enantioselective of ferrugine and its analogues. Tetrahedron. 2012;68:8236-8244

[44] Singh S. Chemistry design, and structure-activity relationship of cocaine antagonists. Chemical Reviews. 2000;100:925-1024

[45] Zakusov VV, Kostochka LM, Skoldinov AP. Effect of cocaine molecule fragments on the central nervous system. Biulleten' Eksperimental'noĭ Biologii i Meditsiny. 1978;86(10):435-438

[46] Takahashi T, Hagi T, Kitano K, Takeuchi Y. 1,3-dipolar cycloaddition of 1-methyl-3-oxidopyridinium and sulfonylethenes. A synthesis of 2-tropanols and monofluorinated 2-tropanol. Chemistry Letters. 1989;18: 593-596. DOI: 10.1246/cl.1989.593

[47] Ronald WW, El-Fawal HAN, John FG, Lung CC, Tali S. Anhydroecogonine compounds and their use as anticholinergic agents. Us 582149 A; 13 October 1998

[48] Gino RT, Burtan MB. Anticholinergic compound. Us 4467095 A; 21 August 1984

[49] Lazer ES, Aggarwal ND, Hite GJ, Neiforth KA, Kelleher RT, Spealman RD, et al. Synthesis and biological activity of cocaine analogs I: N-alkylated norcocaine derivatives. Journal of Pharmaceutical Sciences. 1978;67:1656-1658. DOI: 10.1002/jps.2600671204

[50] Atkinson ER, Mcritchie DD. The Journal of Organic Chemistry. 1971;36: 3240

[51] Grundmann C, Ottmann G. Ein Neuer Synthetischer Weg In Die Tropan-Reihe. European Journal of Organic Chemistry. 1957;605:24-32. DOI: 10.1002/jlac.19576050105

[52] Kyoko O, Osamu I. Process for synthesizing anhydroecyonine derivative. Us 6596868 B2; 22 July 2003

[53] Bell MR, Archer S. Journal of the American Chemical Society. 1958;80:6149

[54] Hobson JD, Bastable JW, Dunkin IR. Solvolytic rearrangements of azabicyclic

compounds. Part 2. Kinetics. Journal of
the Chemical Society, Perkin
Transactions 1. 1981:1346-1351. DOI:
10.1039/P19810001346

[55] Kyoko O, Osamu I. Reacting a
cycloheptatriene derivative with a
primary amine or ammonia in presence
of bas. Us 0020096 A1; 2001

[56] Alsamarrai ASH, Hobson JD.
Synthesis of novel heterocyclic
compounds by nuclophilic addition
reaction of nitrogen nuclophilic to
2-cycloheptatrienylphosphonium
fluoroborate, Jordan. Journal of Applied
Sciences. 2000;**2**(3):56-64

[57] Alsamarrai ASH. Synthesis of
2-(*p*-toluenesulphonyl) tropane-2-ene:
Anhydroecgonine analog. 2017;**192**:
252-254. DOI: 10.1080/
10426507.2016.1252363

Chapter 4

Food Glycoalkaloids: Distribution, Structure, Cytotoxicity, Extraction, and Biological Activity

Md Abu Bakar Siddique and Nigel Brunton

Abstract

Glycoalkaloids (GA), generally occur as plant steroidal glycosides, are secondary metabolites produced in the leaves, flowers, roots, and edible parts including sprouts and skin of the plants of *Solanaceae* family. Many of the plants in this family have been stable parts of human diets for centuries, and thus, the occurrence of these compounds has been extensively studied mainly due to concerns regarding their toxicity. GAs are produced by plants as a resistance to challenges such as insects and pests but may also produce concentration-dependent toxic effects in humans. Postharvest conditions such as light, temperature, humidity, and processing conditions may also affect GA content in edible plants producing them. Since these compounds also possess biological properties such as anti-inflammatory, antimicrobial, and anticarcinogenic activities, it could be a useful strategy to use novel extraction techniques to maintaining bioactivities after extraction and simultaneously to reduce toxicity in the source plants. This chapter aims to describe alkaloids especially GAs commonly occurring in foods, their structure and toxicity, and postharvesting practices which influence alkaloid content and utilization of conventional and novel technologies to extract food alkaloids.

Keywords: food glycoalkaloids, aglycones, α-solamargine, α-solasonine, solasodine, α-chaconine, α-solanine, solanidine, α-tomatine, tomatidine, cytotoxicity, food safety, anticancer, novel technologies

1. Introduction

Plant uses complex biochemical pathways to produce secondary metabolites to tackle adverse environmental stimuli such as damages from herbivores, pathogens, or deprivation of nutrients. These secondary metabolites can be species- or genera-specific and generally do not serve any role in the growth and development of the plants but improve plant viability by increasing their overall ability to cope with the local environmental challenges [1]. Apart from protecting the plant from bacteria, fungi, and viruses, some of the secondary metabolites function as radical-scavenging, UV light-absorbing, and antiproliferative agents [2]. Plants produce a large number of secondary metabolites which, based on their biosynthetic origins, are divided into three major groups: terpenoids, phenolic compounds, and alkaloids [3].

Among plant secondary metabolites, GAs are interesting not only for chemical and biological reasons, but also because they have exerted an important influence on various aspects of human activity and behavior [4]. GAs are steroidal alkaloids that usually possess a sterol skeleton in six heterocyclic rings with a nitrogen. These GAs work as a part of the defense system in many plants including widely consumed agricultural plants of *Solanaceae* family such as potato (*Solanum tuberosum*), tomato (*Solanum lycopersicum*), and aubergine (*Solanum melongena*). Solanine was considered the only compound of this type present in potatoes until chaconine was discovered in 1854. Tomatine, which was in fact the mixture of

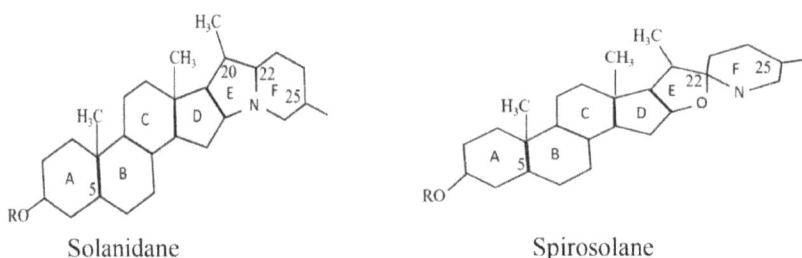

Figure 1.
Structures of solanidane and spirosolane glycoalkaloids (taken from [4]).

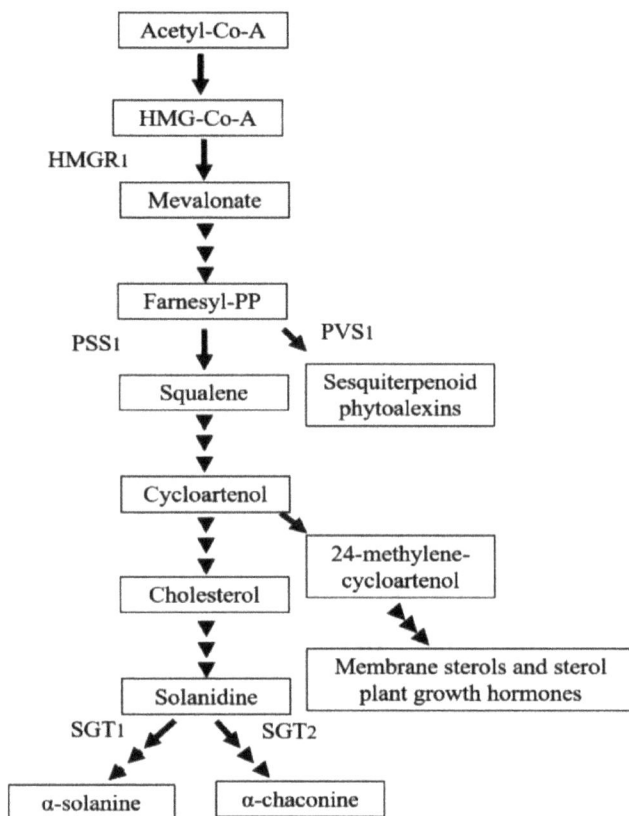

Figure 2.
Schematic representation of proposed steroidal GA biosynthesis. Triple arrowheads represent several enzymatic steps (taken from [11]).

tomatine and dehydrotomatine, was discovered in tomato in 1948. The major GAs of aubergine, solasonine, and solamargine were discovered later and found in 100 other species [5].

Plants often contain alkaloids in glycosidic form as GAs. GAs consist of two structural components: an aglycone structure which is based on C27 cholestane skeleton with an additional nitrogen-containing rings that impart the basicity and oligosaccharide moiety making GAs amphiphatic in nature. The aglycones are divided into five different categories depending on their structure: solanidanes (with fused indolizidine rings), spirosolanes (with an oxa-azaspirodecane alkaloid portion) [6, 7], epiminocholestanes, α-epiminocyclohemiketals, and 3-aminospi-rostanes [8]. Based on the skeletal type of the aglycone, plant steroidal GAs vary as spirosolan types, similar to spirostan, but with nitrogen in place of the oxygen in ring F and another is the solanidane type, where nitrogen connects spirostan rings E and F (**Figure 1**) [9]. At least, 90 structurally unique steroidal alkaloids have been identified in over 350 *Solanum* species. Nitrogen can be attached as a primary NH_2 group in position 3 or 20 (free or methylated), forming simple steroidal bases (e.g., conessine), ring-closed to skeletal or side-chain carbon (as a secondary NH), or annelated in two rings as a tertiary N (e.g., solanidine). This often influences the chemical character of the compound [10]. In addition, a significant portion of the biological activity of GAs derives from the oligosaccharide moieties [4].

Relatively, little is known about the biosynthetic pathway of steroidal glycoalka-loids and the factors that regulate GA levels in plants. However, the aglycone of the steroidal GAs is assumed to be synthesized via the mevalonate/isoprenoid pathway (**Figure 2**). The enzyme 3-hydroxy-3-methylglutaryl coenzyme A reductase (HMGR) catalyzes the first step specific to isoprenoid biosynthesis. Downstream, squalene synthase (PSS1), and vetispiradiene (sesquiterpene) cyclase (PVS1) catalyze the first steps in the branches leading to sterols, steroidal GAs, and sesqui-terpenoid phytoalexins, respectively [11].

2. Distribution of GAs in different plants

2.1 Potato plants

Historically, solanine was the first alkaloid to be isolated from the potatoes [12] and recognized as a glycoside. However, lately, it has been shown that solanine actu-ally was a mixture of two components namely α-solanine and α-chaconine [13]. The two major GAs present in potato (*Solanum tuberosum*), α-solanine and α-chaconine, share the same aglycone, solanidine, but differ with respect to the composition of the sugar side chain (**Figure 3**). α-Chaconine is composed of a branched β-chacotriose (bis-α-L-rhamnopyranosyl-β-D-gluco-pyranose) carbohydrate side chain attached to the 3-OH group of the aglycone, whereas α-solanine has a branched β-solatriose

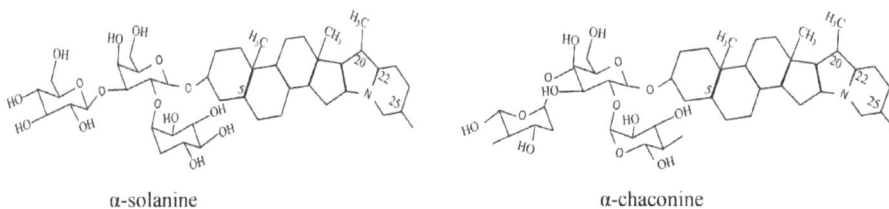

α-solanine   α-chaconine

Figure 3.
Structure of two major GAs from potato (adapted from [5]).

(α-L-rhamnopyranosyl-β-D-glucopyranosyl-β-galactopyranose) side chain also attached to the 3-OH group of the same aglycone. Potatoes may contain small amounts of the hydrolysis products, (β- and γ-chaconines, β- and γ-solanines) solanidine [14].

Apart from commercial varieties α-solanine and α-chaconine, other GAs may also be present in wild species. For example, the leaves and stems of *S. chacoense* contain leptines and leptidines, steroidal alkaloids in addition to the α-solanine and α-chaconine [15]. High levels of GAs are found in potato tissues which undergo intensive metabolic processes, that is, fruits, leaves, stems, tubers eyes, jacket, sprouts, and damaged tissues [16, 17]. While, the GA level associated with the potato sprouts is generally conceded to be higher than that of the rest of the tuber [18]. However, environmental conditions including infection from fungal pathogens and other factors such as climate, soil type, soil moisture, etc., can lead to an increase in the amount of TGA present in any tissue [19]. It has been reported that potato tubers normally contain 1–15 mg/100 g fresh weight of the GAs α-solanine and α-chaconine. Elevated levels of GAs are normally found in potato peels although it should be noted that the peel comprises less than 20% of the total tuber weight [20]. Dao and Friedman [21] used an HPLC assay to determine the amount of α-solanine and α-chaconine in fresh potato leaves at various levels of maturation (from 1 to 9 weeks) in two different potato varieties and found that α-chaconine increased from 20.2 (3 weeks) to 111.4 mg/100 g fresh weight (9 weeks) and α-solanine increased from 9.6 to 50.1 mg/100 g fresh weight over the same period. In another study, Brown et al. [22] showed that the GA content increased with the leaf maturity and then declined with further age when analysis was performed with leaf samples on the same day. Although the amount of GA in potatoes depends on many different factors, **Table 1** gives a good approximation of the ranges that have been reported.

2.2 Tomato plants

About 100 steroidal alkaloids have been found in different tissues and development stages of the tomato plant [24–26]. Tomato plants (*S. lycopersicum*) contain the spirosolane-type GAs α-tomatine and dehydrotomatine (**Figure 4**). The presence of a double bond in the steroidal ring B in structure of dehydrotomatine is the distinguishable feature between α-tomatine and dehydrotomatine. Both of the GAs

Potato part	Total GAs (mg/kg fresh weight)
Tuber with skin	75
Tuber with skin (bitter taste)	250–800
Peel (skin)	150–600
Peel (skin) from bitter tuber	1500–2200
Tuber without skin	12–50
Sprouts	2000–4000
Flower	3000–5000
Stems	30
Leaves	400–1000
Taken from [23].	

Table 1.
Distribution of GA in potatoes.

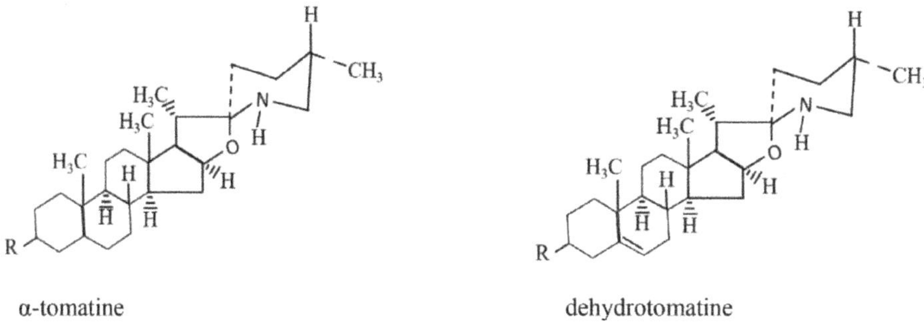

Figure 4.
Structure of α-tomatine and dehydrotomatine (taken from [28]).

have same tetrasaccharide side chain (lycotetraose), but they differ in the aglycone structure. α-Tomatine has lycotetraose attached to the aglycone tomatidine, whereas dehydrotomatine has lycotetraose attached to the aglycone tomatidenol [27].

All parts of the tomato plant including leaves, stems, and tomato fruits contain tomatine and dehydrotomatine. Immature green tomatoes contain up to 500 mg α-tomatine/kg of fruit weight. However, tomatine is largely degraded as the fruit ripens, to a level of only 5 mg/kg of fresh fruit weight in red tomatoes [29]. While unripe green tomatoes contain tomatine and dehydrotomatine, isolation of another major spirosolane-type glycoside esculeoside from mature cherry tomato has also been reported by Fujiwara et al. [30]. However, these authors concluded that esculeosides A and B might be produced from the tomatine in the immature tomato as tomato matures. Again, a wide range of levels of GAs have been reported in the different parts of the tomato plant; however, **Table 2** presents a good approximation of the levels reported.

2.3 Eggplants

Solasonine and solamargine are two major steroidal alkaloids found in eggplant (*Solanum melongena*) (**Figure 5**). These two GAs have the same aglycone (solasodine), but differ in the nature of the trisaccharide side chain. The trisaccharide side chain of solasonine is solatriose, whereas chacotriose is the trisaccharide attached to

Tomato plant part	Dehydrotomatine (mg/kg fresh weight)	α-Tomatine (mg/kg fresh weight)
Large immature green fruit	14	144
Small immature green fruit	54	465
Roots	33	118
Calyxes	62	795
Leaves	71	975
Small stems	138	896
Large stems	142	465
Flowers	190	1100
Senescent leaves	330	4900
Adapted from [5].		

Table 2.
Distribution of GA in tomato fruits and plants.

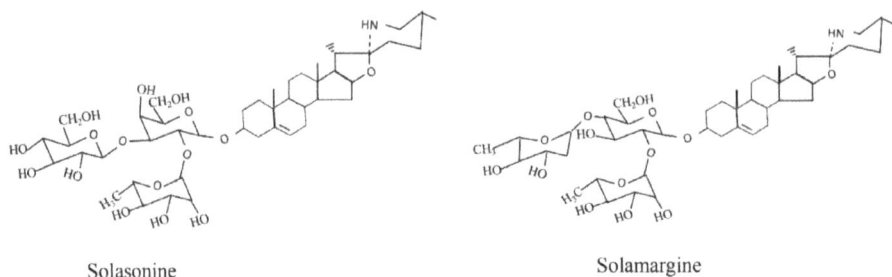

Solasonine　　　　　　　　　　　　　　　　　Solamargine

Figure 5.
Chemical structure of solasonine and solamargine (taken from [34]).

the solasodine aglycone of solamargine [31]. Eggplant GAs differ from those found in major potato alkaloids (α-chaconine and α-solanine) only in the structure of the steroidal part of the molecules, while having identical carbohydrate side chains attached to the aglycone structure. Generally, the GAs solamargine and solasonine are found in the fruits of eggplant. A study of 10 eggplant lines and the 3 allied species (*S. aethiopicum*, *S. integrifolium*, and *S. sodomaeum*) confirmed that the allied species had higher GA content than the widely consumed eggplants and that the GA content generally increased during fruit development and ripening [32]. A calorimetric study of 21 different varieties of *S. melongena* as carried out by Bajaj et al. showed GA content ranged from 6.25 to 20.5 mg/100 g fresh weight (mean value 11.3 mg/100) [33].

3. Human and animal toxicity

None of the *Solanace*ous crops consumed as vegetables are toxic if standard cultivation/production practices are adhered to. However, factors associated with the growth, harvest, and postharvest practices, high temperatures, and wounding may elevate GAs to toxic levels [35]. Several other environmental stresses as well as maturity level and the use of fertilizer can also influence the amount of GA [18]. For example, a significant increase in GA concentration has been reported in potatoes cultivated in drought stress conditions where average concentration increases of 43 and 50% were reported in the improved and control cultivars, respectively [36]. Unusually, cold and wet conditions during potato tuber development and growth have often been assumed as a cause of high glycoalkaloid levels [37]. However, hot and dry conditions during plant growth have also been suggested to be responsible for increasing glycoalkaloid concentrations [38, 39]. It is important for human safety to keep steroidal GA levels as low as possible in edible organs of these crops [16]. Some of the toxic effects of GAs are attributed to direct inhibition of cholinesterase activity and more general cell membrane disruption mediated via interactions between membrane sterols and the steroidal moiety of the steroidal GAs [40–42]. Furthermore, interactions between membrane budding and increased permeability may result in a loss of ion conductivity of the cells [43, 44]. Excessive consumption induces gastroenteritis, gastrointestinal discomfort, diarrhea, vomiting, fever, low blood pressure, fast pulse rate along with neurological and occasional death in human and farm animals [45].

The toxicity of solanine depends on the species and route of administration. Parenteral administration is much more toxic than oral administration. Gastrointestinal effects may occur at relatively low levels of exposure such as lower than 2 mg total GA/kg body weight. The biological half-life of α-solanine is about

21 h; it disrupts the membrane of red blood cells and other cellular membranes and exhibits poor absorption in the gastrointestinal tract, its highest distribution is in spleen, but levels in blood become greatest after about 5 h [46, 47]. Therefore, accumulation of GAs in the body may occur which eventually can lead to adverse health effects [47]. Patil et al. reported that i.p. administration of α-solanine to mice induced irritation for about 1 min and the animals were quiet and appeared to be sleepy and apathetic, exhibiting more rapid breathing, hind leg paralysis, and dyspnea [48]. While α-chaconine is considered more toxic than α-solanine, a combination of both of these GAs can induce a synergistic toxic effect. α-Chaconine has a half-life of about 44 h, longer than that of α-solanine [47]. In mice, the i.p. LD_{50} was reported to be 27.5 mg/kg, and in rabbits, the lowest lethal dose was 50 mg/kg i.p. [49].

Although tomatine also alters cell membranes [50], its oral toxicity is low when compared to other GAs, presumably because its cholesterol complex is not absorbed from the gut [51]. The amount of α-tomatine in the tubers of somatic hybrids in tomato and potato has been reported to be 5- to 10-fold higher than those in their parents [52], and these levels could pose a health threat if consumed by humans. Unripe green tomatoes are routinely consumed as fried vegetables or as pickles, and fruits "turning" from green to red are preferred raw by some consumers. Overconsumption of such fruit poses a potential health risk due to α-tomatine toxicity [16]. According to Roddick, lethality occurred within 0.5–2 min in mice, to which α-tomatine was administrated intravenously at a level of 18 mg/kg of body weight. The most common responses to intravenous α-tomatine administration are a large decrease in blood pressure and fluctuations in respiratory rate. Where the dose of α-tomatine was lethal, death was thought to be due to a drop in blood pressure, but with sublethal doses, the initial drop was followed by an equally rapid recovery [53].

Only a few studies concerning the toxicity of solamargine have been published. However, a study conducted by Zheng et al. reported that the biotransformation of solamargine is relatively quick. Eight hours after an intravenous administration of 4 mg/kg to rats, only a trace amount of solamargine could be detected [54].

4. Postharvest technologies that influence the amount of GAs

A number of factors influence the formation of GA's preharvest, during harvest, and postharvest. These factors can be summarized as follows:

1. potato cultivars and environmental and growing conditions;

2. maturity during harvesting time, temperature during growth, and extent of sprouting;

3. any mechanical damage such as bruising, cutting, wounding, and slicing that has occurred during handling;

4. postharvest storage conditions in particular wavelength, duration, and intensity of light during storage;

5. other environmental conditions during packaging, transportation, and marketing [55–57].

Considerable research has been performed on potato storage conditions such as temperature, time, and light, and it has been found that these conditions have a profound impact on the GA level of potatoes. Scientific reports on the effect of temperature on potato GAs are however somewhat conflicting. For example, one study reported a twofold higher level of GA in potato tubers after 6 weeks storage at 4–6°C compared to those stored at 12–15°C [58]. The amount of GA has also been reported to increase at 10°C, while further decreasing the temperature to 4.4°C resulted in only a minor change [59]. A rise in the solanine content in tubers stored at high temperatures was also reported by Salunkhe et al., who found small increase in potato stored at 0 and 8°C and much greater increase in those stored at 15 and 24°C. These authors concluded that the increase may be related to a stress response [60].

The amount of GAs can also vary as a result of exposure to varying light sources such as daylight, UV, fluorescent, and incandescent light during harvesting, storage, and transportation [61]. For example, Machado et al. investigated the effect of different light sources and temperature on the level of GAs in potato tubers. Their investigation involved exposing potato tubers (cv Monaliza) to a range of conditions such as indirect sunlight, fluorescent light, storage in darkness under refrigeration, and storage in darkness at room temperature for 14 days. Potato tubers exposed to fluorescent light had the highest GA levels. Increases in GA levels in lower size potato tubers stored under indirect sunlight and fluorescent light were approximately 4–6 times greater than that of potato tubers stored in darkness at room temperature [58]. Similarly, Salunkhe et al. reported that exposure to sunlight or artificial light can increase GA synthesis in potatoes by factors of 3 or 4 compared to those of potatoes stored in the dark [60]. Other authors have reported that the blue spectral portion (<500 nm, especially UV light <300 nm) and infrared light (1300 nm) are active elicitors of GAs synthesis; while light of 570–700 nm enhances chlorophyll but not GA synthesis [62]. For storing potatoes for a longer period, it is necessary to choose unwounded and ungreened potatoes, and to store in the dark at 5–8°C to prevent sprouting and a corresponding increase in GA content.

It has been reported that domestic cooking and processing such as boiling, baking, and frying does not reduce the amount of GAs in potatoes. The cooking of potatoes has variable effects since GAs are very heat stable, with solanine decomposing at temperatures between 260 and 270°C [63]. While boiling of potatoes does not affect the level of GAs, there are some reports that microwaving could reduce this amount. For example, in a study conducted by Takagi et al., a reduction of alkaloid content by 15% was reported following microwaving, whereas boiling lowered the α-chaconine and α- solanine content by 3.5 and 1.2%, respectively [64]. However, since GAs are localized near the skin (usually no deeper than 3 mm), peeling deep enough to remove any green layer will remove most of the GAs [65]. In most potatoes, the peel contains 60–80% of GAs [66], while for bitter-tasting potatoes, this amount was found to be 30–35% [67]. Generally, chips and fries are considered to be nonhazardous as processing involves the removal of the peel of the potatoes. Potatoes are a versatile commodity and this is reflected in the range of products for which GA levels have been measured by other authors as presented in **Table 3**.

Generally, tomatine is quite stable in food; studies, however, have shown that some products based on unripe green tomatoes lost a considerable amount of tomatine during prolonged storage [69, 70]. Cooking for a shorter time (5 min) had a marginal effect, while considerable losses of tomatine (90–95%) were observed during storage of freeze-dried products at room temperature for 4 weeks, the loss being greater for whole tomatoes than for pulp [69]. Storing green tomato fruits, containing 90 mg tomatine/kg of fresh weight (1040 mg/kg dry weight), for up to 170 days at −20°C as a freeze-dried product, after pulping and sterilization at 121°C for 30 min, and preserved with benzoic acid resulted in an increase in the content of tomatine for all products during the first week of storage and a decrease thereafter. After 50 and 170 days storing, the content of tomatine was reduced to

Product of preparation	GA concentration (mg/kg product)
Boiled peeled potato[a]	27–42
Baked jacket potato[a]	99–113
Chips (US: French fries)	0.4–8
Chips (UK)	19–58
Oven chips (UK)	27–86
Fried skins	567–1450
Frozen mashed potato	2–5
Frozen baked potato	80–123
Frozen chips	2–29
Part cooked frozen chips	23–55
Precooked frozen chips	19–35
Frozen skins	65–121
Frozen fried potato	4–31
Canned peeled potato	1–2
Canned whole new potato (tubers)	24–34
Canned whole new potato (liquor)	15–17
Canned potato (UK)	29–99
Crisps (US: potato chips)	23–180
Crisps (UK: potato chips)	32–184
Crisps (Norwich)	59–70
Crisps (with skin)	95–720
Dehydrated potato flour	65–75
Potato powder	39–135
Dehydrated potato flakes	15–23

Taken from [68].

[a]Noncommercial preparation.

Table 3.
Levels of GA in various commercial potato products and preparations.

around 60 and 20 mg/kg dry weight in all products [70]. In a review, Friedman and Levine mentioned the average amount of α-tomatine present in a half-cup (125 g) of condensed tomato soup, one table spoon of ketchup (15 g), and 6 fl oz. (183 g) of juice as 0.2, 0.13, and 0.5 (mg)/serving, respectively. Other tomato products, such as half fruit of green pickled (40 g), contain 2.9 mg, while 133 g of fried green tomato contains 1.5 mg of tomatine/serving size [71].

5. Anticancer activity

The ability of SGAs to disrupt cellular structure has been examined by some researchers as a possible application of these compounds for treating cancer cells. Extracts obtained from *Solanum* spp. have been used to treat cancer for centuries and there are some indications that they possess cytotoxic activity. For example, α-solanine was found to have a proliferation-inhibiting and an apoptosis-promoting effect on multiple cancer cells, such as clone, liver, melanoma cancer cells [72]. Friedman et al. [73] examined the impact of GAs extracted from one potato variety and mixtures of GAs extracted from five different widely consumed commercial potato varieties in Korea and Japan on a number of cancer cell lines. They reported a reduction in the numbers of the following cell lines: cervical (HeLa), liver (HepG2), lymphoma (U937), stomach (AGS and KATO III) cancer cells, and normal liver cells and that this effect was concentration dependent (0.1–10 µg/ml) with α-chaconine being more effective than α-solanine. Ji et al. observed induction of apoptosis in the HepG2 cell line from the digestive tracts using the MTT assay and screening the sensitive cells and then measuring the morphological changes of the tumor cells. These authors observed that sub-G_0 apoptosis peaks at different doses of solanine and that a decrease in the content of antiapoptotic protein was dose dependent. In pancreatic cancer cells, a nontoxic quantity of solanine (3, 6, and 9 µg/µl) inhibited metastasis (*in vitro*), such as invasion, migration, and angiogenesis, which demonstrated that the inhibitory effect of solanine on metastasis was via its cytotoxic activity. In these cancer cells, α-solanine stimulated p53 and Bax but also suppressed Bcl-2, which led to a release of cytochrome *c* within the mitochondrial pathway of apoptosis. The decrease in Bcl-2 and increase in Bax were also demonstrated in cancer tissue [74]. An increase in proapoptotic Bax protein in breast cancer tissue in mice treated with α-solanine was shown by Mohsenikia et al. [75].

However, several other studies have shown that α-solanine can lead to cancer development and metastasis suppression through inhibition of vascular endothelial growth factor (VEGF) and matrix metalloproteinases (MMPs) [76]. MMPs are believed to participate in tumor cell migration, tissue invasion, and metastasis [77]. In another study, Pan et al. noted α-solanine-induced prostate cancer cell inhibition through the suppression of cell cyclin proteins and through the induction of reactive oxygen species and activation of P38 MAPK pathway [78]. Another effect of α-solanine in cancer cells is the inhibition of cell migration and invasion caused by inhibition of the phosphorylation of JNK, PI3 K, and Akt and, thus, the inhibition of MMP-2 and -9 expressions. In addition, a downregulation of the nuclear content of NF-κB was demonstrated in α-solanine-treated cells [79]. Furthermore, Lee et al. investigated the role of potato GAs such as α-chaconine and solanine and their hydrolysis products at four concentrations (0.1, 1, 10, and 100 µg/mL) on the human colon (HT-29) and liver (Hep G2) cell lines. Results showed that α-chaconine was more effective on both of the cell lines, the inhibition of both cell lines increased with the concentration but did not appear to be in a linear function of the concentration and the inhibition of the liver cells was greater than that of colon cells. The hydrolysis product of α-chaconine, that is, γ-chaconine exhibited low activity against the colon cells in contrast to the high activity against the liver cells. The activity of γ-chaconine against the liver cells was greater than those mentioned for *β1*- and *β2*-chaconine and approached that of α-chaconine. In the case of α-solanine, the inhibitory activity at the 100 µg/mL level was similar for both cell lines and the inhibition at a reduced concentration was lower than that of α-chaconine. These results suggest that the nature and presence of the carbohydrate moiety can affect cytotoxicity [80].

Recently, the anticancer effect of α-tomatine and its mechanism of action have been studied. It has been proposed that tomatine can kill cells by binding to cell membranes followed by leakage of cell components [81]. Binding of tomatine to cholesterol may be relevant to the mechanism of inhibition of carcinogenesis. Despite the ability to disrupt cell membranes *in vitro*, orally consumed tomatine is not toxic, presumably because it forms an insoluble complex with cholesterol in the digestive tract, which is then eliminated in the faces [82]. In addition, Sucha et al. observed an inhibition in MCF-7 human breast adenocarcinoma cell line proliferation and viability at α-tomatine concentrations from 6 to 9 µM and postulated that the cytotoxic mechanism could be due the fact that cholesterol in biological membranes serves as a target for the α-tomatine [83]. It has also been reported that α-tomatine suppresses cell adhesion, morphology/actin cytoskeleton arrangement, invasion and migration in human nonsmall cell lung cancer NCI-H460 cells. The authors compared of 0 μM, after 24 and 48 h treatment with tomatine at a concentration between 0 and 1.5 μM and reported no significant alteration of cell viability, indicating that the compound is not toxic to NCI-H460 at these dosages. However, cell viability was significantly decreased when the applied concentration of tomatine was increased to 2–4 μM for 24 and 48 h [84]. Furthermore, α-tomatine induced a significant cytotoxic effect on the human leukemia cancer cell line HL60 and K562. Experiments using the MTT assay revealed that tomatine has strong cytotoxic effect that could inhibit cell survival of HL60 and K562 in a concentration-dependent manner with an IC_{50} of 1.92 and 1.51 μM, respectively. According to Chao et al., cancer cells exposed to tomatine led to a loss of the mitochondrial membrane potential and triggered the release of the apoptosis-inducing factor (AIF) from the mitochondria into the nucleus and downregulated surviving expression [85]. In addition, Rudolf and Rudolf [86] also noted the cytotoxic effect of tomatine on human colon cancer cells was related to lysosomal membrane permeabilization including mitochondrial perturbation with subsequent mitochondrial release of apoptosis-inducing factor (AIF) that contributed to the execution of diverse death phenotypes, possibly via enhanced activity of JNK but in the absence of significant oxidative stress. In another recent study, the effect of tomatine separately and in combination with curcumin on the growth and apoptosis of human prostate cancer PC-3 cell was investigated [87]. In this study, authors reported that a low concentration of both anticancer agents did not have any impact separately, while the combination of these anticancer agents (1 μM tomatine and 5 μM curcumin) synergistically inhibited the growth of cultured prostate cancer cells, mainly associated with inhibition of NF-κB activation and decreased levels of Bcl-2, phospho-Akt, and phospho-ERK1/2. The hydrolysates such as β1 tomatine, γ-tomatine, δ-tomatine, and their common aglycone are reported to have lower activity on the cancer cells than α-tomatine [80, 88].

Like other steroidal GAs, solamargine has been reported to inhibit the growth of human cancer cells, for example, colon (HT-29 and HCT-15), prostate (LNCaP and PC-3), breast (T47D and MDA-MB-231), human hepatoma (PLC/PRF/5), and JTC-26 cells [89, 90]. However, the molecular mechanisms underlying the effect of solamargine to inhibit the growth and induce apoptosis of various cancer cells are poorly understood. Solamargine inhibits proliferation and induces apoptosis in lung cancer cells through p38 MAPK-mediated suppression of phosphorylation and protein expression of Stat3, followed by inducing Stat3 downstream effector p21 [90]. Another study showed that solamargine inhibits the growth of human lung cancer cells through reduction of EP4 protein expression, followed by increasing ERK1/2 phosphorylation [91]. Shiu et al. demonstrated solamargine had a greater cytotoxic effect than cisplatin, methotrexate, 5-fluorouracil, epirubicin, and cyclophosphamide against human breast cancer cell lines. In this study, the authors demonstrated that solamargine upregulated the expressions of external death receptors, such as tumor necrosis factor receptor I (TNFR-I), Fas receptor (Fas), TNFR-I-associated death domain (TRADD), and Fas-associated death domain (FADD). Solamargine also enhanced the intrinsic ratio of Bax to Bcl-2 by upregulating Bax and downregulating Bcl-2 and Bcl-xL expressions. Ultimately, the effects, induced by solamargine, released mitochondrial cytochrome c and activation of caspase-8, -9, and -3 in the cells, indicating that solamargine triggered extrinsic and intrinsic apoptotic pathways to breast cancer cells [92]. Furthermore, no cell cycle arrest was observed in the human myelogenous leukemia K562 cell line, but cytotoxicity to different human cancer cell lines was reported. Solamargine caused membrane disruption and blebbing independent of calcium, and a decrease in ATP levels. These changes are typical in oncosis, the process leading to necrotic cell death [93–95]. The carbohydrate moiety of solamargine significantly affects its anticancer activity. Considering the difference of the -L-rhamnopyranosyl-(12) between solamargine and khasianine (**Figure 6**), Chang et al. found that the cell death by apoptosis between these two was significantly different. The IC_{50} (dose that inhibits cell growth by 50%) of solamargine, solasodine, and khasianine were 3.0, 2.7, and greater than 20 g/ml, respectively [96].

Furthermore, anticancer properties of solasodine in a mice model were investigated in vivo and it was shown that solasodine glycoside treatments exerted significant inhibition of murine sarcoma 180 cell lines (S180) [97]. Based on further molecular investigation, the probable role of rhamnose in solasodine glycosides binding on tumor cells and its specificity was proposed. About 0.005% mixture of solasodine glycosides (Zycure) was demonstrated to be an effective dose on human beings. About 0.005% exhibited 66 and 78% curability at 56 days and 1 year follow-up, respectively [98]. The possibility of using these GAs from the same and/or different food sources and with other therapeutic agents additively or synergistically has also been taken under consideration. According to Roddick and Rijnenberg, synergism between solanine and chaconine in relation to their membrane-lytic action appeared to be a real and potentially important phenomenon. The two major potato GAs had a significantly greater effect on phosphatidylcholine/cholesterol liposomes at pH 7.2 when used in combination as compared to separately. The latter imparted little or no effect at concentrations up to 1 mM but the former caused greater membrane disruption and leakage of entrapped content at about 100 μM or less [99]. The maximum synergistic effect on C6 rat glioma cells was observed at a ratio 1:1 between α-solanine and α-chaconine at micromolar concentrations [100]. Friedman et al. demonstrated inhibition of liver and stomach cancer cell growth after treatment with α-solanine or α-chaconine alone or in combination. The combination of these two compounds exerted a synergistic, additive, or antagonistic effect on the investigated cell lines [73]. On the other hand, evidence showed that solamargine can be used in combination with some cancer drugs including methotrexate, 5-florouracil, cisplatin, and epirubicin to improve effectiveness on several cancer cell lines and may have potential in breast and lung cancer therapies [92, 101–103]. Furthermore, studies suggest that the combinations of lycopene and α-tomatine, both in pure form and in red and in green tomatoes and tomato products, can have health-improving benefits at lower concentrations than of each bioactive compound alone. Studies suggest that both lycopene and α-tomatine might contribute to the prevention and therapy for human cancers and possibly also cardiovascular diseases [27].

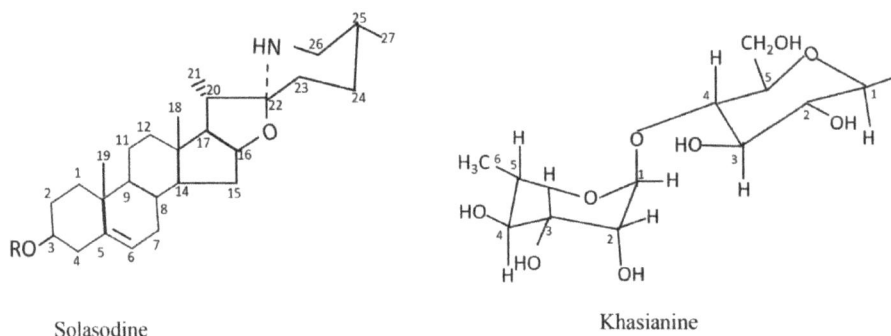

Solasodine

Khasianine

Figure 6.
Structure of solasodine and khasianine (taken from [96]).

6. Antifungal, antimicrobial, and insecticidal activity

In plants, GAs have antimicrobial, insecticidal, and fungicidal properties which account for their protective activity against several insect, pests, and herbivores. α-Chaconine and α-solanine and various *Solanum* sp. extracts have been shown to be toxic to leaf-eating insects, pests of stored products (e.g., seed and flour), mosquitos that feed on animal tissues, termites and cockroaches that feed on feces and garbage, and predatory species [104]. In a recent study, Friedman et al. reported that the GAs α-chaconine and α-solanine were highly active against three pathogenic strains of trichomonads. These authors also reported that the activity of α-solanine was several times higher than α-chaconine; which is contrary to the several previous results where the influence of α-chaconine was reported higher than that of α-solanine [105]. Several other research works regarding the impact of potato glycoalkaloids on the membrane of frog embryos [106–108] and on fungi such as *A. crenulatus*, *A. brassicicola*, *P. medicaginis*, and *R. solani* [109, 110] showed that α-chaconine was more active than α-solanine. Therefore, it appears that the configuration and/or content of the sugar moieties of the molecules influence activity. It has also been reported that the synergism of the two major GAs significantly delivers greater membrane-disruptive activity than either alone. As for example, Fewell and Roddick observed that administration of solanine alone resulted in a minor inhibition in *A. brassicicola* and *P. medicaginis* spore germination; however, significant enhancement in inhibition was observed upon coadministration with α-chaconine [111]. On the other hand, Dahlin et al. showed that α-solanine and α-chaconine exert no significant direct inhibition of mycelial growth of *P. infestans*, while the nonglycosylated unit solanidine has a strong inhibitory effect [112]. It has been reported that the impact of glycoalkaloids on fungi depends not only on the GA structure but also on the species, culture conditions, and development stages of the fungus [111]. Some published reports have indicated the possible use of crude potato extract as an insecticidal source. For instance, Nenaah reported that both potato extract and GAs exhibited considerable acute and residual toxicity against adults of the red flour beetle *Tribolium castaneum* Herbst and the rice weevil *Sitophilus oryzae* L. in a dose-depending manner, but potato extract was more toxic than pure GAs [113]. Moreover, the bactericidal effect of freeze-dried potato peel extract was investigated for mutagenic activity using *in vitro Salmonella typhimurium-Escherichia coli* microsome assay by Stillo et al. These authors, however, proposed that the impact was only significant when used at a higher concentration (100,000 g/ml) [114]. The antibacterial properties of potato peel extract also vary with the species of microorganism examined. For example, Amanpour et al. reported that an ethanol extract from the peel of *Solanum tuberosum* had an antibacterial effect on a spectrum of Gram-positive bacteria, particularly on *S. aureus* but was only effective on one Gram-negative bacteria namely *P. aeruginosa* [115].

Tomato GAs also protect plants against insects and fungal plant pathogens and act by disrupting cell membranes by lysing liposomes [71]. Previously, Roddick [53] reported that a tomatine concentration of 10–30 mg/kg was high enough to be toxic to several fungal species. α-Tomatine has been shown to kill a broad range of fungi and functions as a resistant substance against phytopathogens in the tomato plant [116]. Sandrock and VanEtten examined the impact of α-tomatine on 23 fungal strains and found that both saprophytes and all five pathogens which are nontoxic to tomato were highly sensitive, while all but two tomato pathogens (*Stemphylium solani* and *Verticillium dahliae*) were tolerant to this toxic compound (50% effective dose >300 μM). These authors also tested the sensitivity of the fungal isolates to the hydrolysis products of α-tomatine (β2 tomatine and tomatidine) and found them to be less toxic to most pathogens but inhibitory to some of the saprophytes and nonpathogens of tomato [116]. According to several other published results, the hydrolysis products of tomatines possess reduced antifungal activity [43, 117]. In fact, it has been previously reported that fungal tomato pests such as *Septoria lycopersici* and *Fusarium oxysporum* have been found to produce extracellular enzymes that hydrolyze glycosidic bonds within the saccharide chain of α-tomatine, which not only exhibit reduced antifungal activity but also cause suppression of induced plant defense mechanisms such as hypersensitive responses and oxidative burst [117, 118]. Furthermore, a preliminary screening showed that tomatine at a concentration of 100 μM completely inhibited the growth of the *Trichomonas vaginalis* strain G3, *Tritrichomonas foetus* strain D1, and *Tritrichomonas foetus* strain C1, while much less inhibition was found in the case of tomatidine [119]. However, in contrast, Simons et al. found that the aglycone tomatidine has far more antifungal activity toward yeast and a more distinct mode of action than α-tomatine [120]. The membrane lytic effect of α-tomatine is pH dependent, and it has also mentioned that some fungi are able to colonize α-tomatine-containing tomato tissue by lowering the pH of the infection site [121].

Like other steroidal GAs, there is also some evidence that solasonine and solamargine possess antifungal, insecticidal, and molluscicidal activities. Both glycoalkaloids are reported to inhibit growth of the spiny bollworm, lettuce seedlings, and molluscs, while solasonine is weakly antiviral [122–126]. The antifungal activity has also been reported for solamargine and to a lesser extent for its aglycone solasodine [127, 128]. Furthermore, inhibition of red flour beetle larvae, tobacco hornworms, and *Trypanosoma cruzi* by solamargine has been reported [128, 129].

7. Other biological activities

In addition to the activities reported above, some GAs have been reported to possess antibiotic, antiallergenic, antipyretic, anti-inflammatory, and anti-hyperglycemic activities at certain doses and conditions. Choi and Koo studied the analgesic and anti-inflammatory effect of a potato extract. They reported that an ethanolic extract of potato resulted in a significant effect in three types of pain induction suggesting that its analgesic effect may in part be related to its anti-inflammatory neurogenic and narcotic properties [130]. The antinociceptive effect of the potato extract may be related to the reduction in Ca^{2+} influx at the axon terminal of the afferent nerve inducing a decrease in adenylyl cyclase activity, which results in decreased levels of cyclic AMP and efflux of K^+ ions. The latter lead to hyperpolarization of the nerve and finally an apparent antinociceptive effect [131]. A recent study highlighted a significant reduction in the production of both proinflammatory cytokines (interleukin-2 and interleukin-8) with sublethal concentrations of α-chaconine (~22% reduction in production of both cytokines) and solanidine (~35% reduction in production of both cytokines) [132]. Shin et al. reported that α-solanine had potential therapeutic value for treatment of inflammatory diseases. The anti-inflammatory effect of solanine was reported to be mediated via the regulation of proinflammatory cytokines in an LPS-induced systemic inflammation mouse model and in RAW 264.7 macrophages [133]. Similarly, tomatine imparted an anti-inflammatory effect to the rats [134]. Although the anti-inflammatory mechanism of α-tomatine is not well understood, results showed that α-tomatine significantly suppressed the production of proinflammatory cytokines in lipopolysaccharide-induced macrophages. Moreover, lipopolysaccharide-mediated nuclear translocation of the nuclear factor-kappa B (NF-κB)-p65 and phosphorylation of extracellular signal-regulated kinase (ERK) 1/2 were attenuated after α-tomatine treatment [135]. In addition, tomatidine exhibited more active anti-inflammatory activity and less toxicity than solasodine. The anti-inflammatory activity of tomatidine is proposed to be due to blocking NF-kB and JNK signaling [136]. The antimalarial activity of chaconine has been reported by Chen et al. Chaconine showed a dose-dependent suppression of malaria infection; at a dose of 7.50 mg/kg, the parasitemia suppressions of chaconine, tomatine, solamargine, solasonine, and solanine were 71.38, 65.25, 64.89, 57.47, and 41.30%, respectively [137]. Furthermore, solanine injected to normal rats increased the blood sugar level, while decreasing of sugar level was observed in case of adrenalectomized rats [138]. Hyperglycemia appears to be due to stimulation of the adrenal gland by solanine. The latter was accompanied by a decrease in glycogen levels in the livers [14]. Another study reported that feeding unripe tomato to the rats significantly reduced blood glucose level compared to the ripe tomatoes, probably due to the presence of large of amount of glycoalkaloids such as tomatine, dehydrotomatine, and tomatidine [139]. On the other hand, it has been reported that a green tomato-rich diet can contribute to cholesterol reduction due to the formation of a complex between α-tomatine and cholesterol [51].

8. Conclusion

In this chapter, information on the distribution of steroidal GAs in the plants of *Solanaceous* family, their harmful effects as well as the beneficial aspects have been reviewed and discussed. GAs are naturally occurring agents which serve a plant protective role in many important commonly consumed plants. Due to their dose-dependent toxicity, excessive accumulation during growth, harvesting, and postharvest practices could lead to the human health problems. On the other hand, if extracted from source, these GAs could be beneficially utilized as insecticide, antimicrobial, and antifungal agents. In recent years, anticancer activity of these compounds has been studied intensively. However, to establish these GAs in cancer treatment, more research works are needed to understand its mechanism and the harmful effects on the normal living cells. In addition, better strategies for recovery of these agents from their natural sources which take account of the need for sustainability need to be further developed. A better understanding of the role of GAs in the plant is also essential to exploit their benefits more effectively by clearly understanding their biological properties which recognizes not only the complexity of living cells, but also the capacity for unique interrelationships between some or all the component compounds.

Author details

Md Abu Bakar Siddique and Nigel Brunton*
Department of Agriculture and Food Science, University College Dublin (UCD)
Belfield, Dublin, Ireland

*Address all correspondence to: nigel.brunton@ucd.ie

IntechOpen

References

[1] Harborne JB. Introduction to Ecological Biochemistry. Academic Press; 2014

[2] Kennedy DO, Wightman EL. Herbal extracts and phytochemicals: Plant secondary metabolites and the enhancement of human brain function. Advances in Nutrition. 2011;**2**(1):32-50. DOI: 10.3945/an.110.000117

[3] Yazaki K. Transporters of secondary metabolites. Current Opinion in Plant Biology. 2005;**8**(3):301-307. DOI: 10.1016/j.pbi.2005.03.011

[4] Roddick JG. Steroidal glycoalkaloids: Nature and consequences of bioactivity. In: Saponins Used in Traditional and Modern Medicine. Boston, MA: Springer; 1996. pp. 277-295

[5] Milner SE, Brunton NP, Jones PW, O'Brien NM, Collins SG, Maguire AR. Bioactivities of glycoalkaloids and their aglycones from *Solanum* species. Journal of Agricultural and Food Chemistry. 2011;**59**(8):3454-3484. DOI: 10.1021/jf200439q

[6] Makkar HP, Norvsambuu T, Lkhagvatseren S, Becker K. Plant secondary metabolites in some medicinal plants of Mongolia used for enhancing animal health and production. Tropicultura. 2009;**27**(3):159-167

[7] Mazid M, Khan T, Mohammad F. Role of secondary metabolites in defense mechanisms of plants. Biology and Medicine. 2011;**3**:232-249

[8] Vaananen T. Glycoalkaloid Content and Starch Structure in Solanum Species and Interspecific Somatic Potato Hybrids. University of Helsinki; 2007

[9] Tek N. Chromatographic Determination of Glycoalkaloids in Eggplant. Izmir Institute of Technology; 2006

[10] Dinan L, Harmatha J, Lafont R. Chromatographic procedures for the isolation of plant steroids. Journal of Chromatography A. 2001;**935**(1-2):105-123. DOI: 10.1016/S0021-9673(01)00992-X

[11] Krits P, Fogelman E, Ginzberg I. Potato steroidal glycoalkaloid levels and the expression of key isoprenoid metabolic genes. Planta. 2007;**227**(1):143-150. DOI: 10.1007/s00425-007-0602-3

[12] Baup S. Extrait d 'une lettre sur plusieurs nouvelles substances. Annales de Chimie Physique. 1826;**31**:108-109

[13] Friedman M, McDonald GM, Filadelfi-Keszi M. Potato glycoalkaloids: Chemistry, analysis, safety, and plant physiology. Critical Reviews in Plant Sciences. 1997;**16**(1):55-132. DOI: 10.1080/07352689709701946

[14] Friedman M. Potato glycoalkaloids and metabolites: Roles in the plant and in the diet. Journal of Agricultural and Food Chemistry. 2006;**54**(23):8655-8681. DOI: 10.1021/jf061471t

[15] Chen Z, Miller AR. Steroidal alkaloids in *Solanaceous* vegetable crops. Horticultural Reviews. 2000;**25**:171-196. DOI: 10.1002/9780470650783.ch3

[16] Percival G, Dixon GR. Glycoalkaloid concentrations in aerial tubers of potato (*Solanum tuberosum* L). Journal of the Science of Food and Agriculture. 1996;**70**(4):439-448. DOI: 10.1002/(SICI)1097-0010(199604)70:43.3.CO;2-8

[17] Pęksa A, Gołubowska G, Rytel E, Lisińska G, Aniołowski K. Influence of harvest date on glycoalkaloid contents of three potato varieties. Food Chemistry. 2002;**78**(3):313-317. DOI: 10.1016/S0308-8146(02)00101-2

[18] Gregory P. Glycoalkaloid composition of potatoes: Diversity and biological implications. American Potato Journal. 1984;**61**(3):115

[19] Maga JA. Potato glycoalkaloids. CRC Critical Reviews in Food Science and Nutrition. 1980;**12**:371-405

[20] Sinden SL, Sanford LL, Webb RE. Genetic and environmental control of potato glycoalkaloids. American Potato Journal. 1984;**61**(3):141

[21] Dao L, Friedman M. Comparison of glycoalkaloid content of fresh and freeze-dried potato leaves determined by HPLC and colorimetry. Journal of Agricultural and Food Chemistry. 1996;**44**(8):2287-2291. DOI: 10.1021/jf9502820

[22] Brown MS, McDonald GM, Friedman M. Sampling leaves of young potato (*Solanum tuberosum*) plants for glycoalkaloid analysis. Journal of Agricultural and Food Chemistry. 1999;**47**(6):2331-2334. DOI: 10.1021/jf981124m

[23] Wood FA, Young DA. TGA in potatoes. Canada Department of Agriculture. 1974;**1533**:1-3

[24] Moco S, Bino RJ, Vorst O, Verhoeven HA, de Groot J, van Beek TA, et al. A liquid chromatography-mass spectrometry-based metabolome database for tomato. Plant Physiology. 2006;**141**(4):1205-1218

[25] Mintz-Oron S, Mandel T, Rogachev I, Feldberg L, Lotan O, Yativ M, et al. Gene expression and metabolism in tomato fruit surface tissues. Plant Physiology. 2008;**147**(2):823-851

[26] Schwahn K, de Souza LP, Fernie AR, Tohge T. Metabolomics-assisted refinement of the pathways of steroidal glycoalkaloid biosynthesis in the tomato clade. Journal of Integrative Plant Biology. 2014;**56**(9):864-875. DOI: 10.1111/jipb.12274

[27] Friedman M. Anticarcinogenic, cardioprotective, and other health benefits of tomato compounds lycopene, α-tomatine, and tomatidine in pure form and in fresh and processed tomatoes. Journal of Agricultural and Food Chemistry. 2013;**61**(40): 9534-9550. DOI: 10.1021/jf402654e

[28] Kozukue N, Han JS, Lee KR, Friedman M. Dehydrotomatine and α-tomatine content in tomato fruits and vegetative plant tissues. Journal of Agricultural and Food Chemistry. 2004;**52**(7):2079-2083. DOI: 10.1021/jf0306845

[29] Friedman M. Analysis of biologically active compounds in potatoes (*Solanum tuberosum*), tomatoes (*Lycopersicon esculentum*), and jimson weed (*Datura stramonium*) seeds. Journal of Chromatography A. 2004;**1054**(1-2):143-155. DOI: 10.1016/j.chroma.2004.04.049

[30] Fujiwara Y, Takaki A, Uehara Y, Ikeda T, Okawa M, Yamauchi K, et al. Tomato steroidal alkaloid glycosides, esculeosides A and B, from ripe fruits. Tetrahedron. 2004;**60**(22):4915-4920

[31] Blankemeyer JT, McWilliams ML, Rayburn JR, Weissenberg M, Friedman M. Developmental toxicology of solamargine and solasonine glycoalkaloids in frog embryos. Food and Chemical Toxicology. 1998;**36**(5):383-389. DOI: 10.1016/S0278-6915(97)00164-6

[32] Mennella G, Lo Scalzo R, Fibiani M, D'Alessandro A, Francese G, Toppino L, et al. Chemical and bioactive quality traits during fruit ripening in eggplant (*S. melongena* L.) and allied species. Journal of Agricultural and Food Chemistry. 2012;**60**(47):11821-11831. DOI: 10.1021/jf3037424

[33] Bajaj KL, Kaur G, Chadha ML. Glycoalkaloid content and other chemical constituents of the

fruits of some egg plant (*Solanum melongena*, L.) varieties. Journal of Plant Foods. 1979;**3**(3):163-168. DOI: 10.1080/0142968X.1979.11904224

[34] Tavares DC, Munari CC, de Freitas Araújo MG, Beltrame MC, Furtado MA, Gonçalves CC, et al. Antimutagenic potential of *Solanum lycocarpum* against induction of chromosomal aberrations in V79 cells and micronuclei in mice by doxorubicin. Planta Medica. 2011;**77**:1489-1494. DOI: 10.1055/s-0030-1270886

[35] Ginzberg I, Tokuhisa JG, Veilleux RE. Potato steroidal glycoalkaloids: Biosynthesis and genetic manipulation. Potato Research. 2009;**52**(1):1-5

[36] Bejarano L, Mignolet E, Devaux A, Espinola N, Carrasco E, Larondelle Y. Glycoalkaloids in potato tubers: The effect of variety and drought stress on the α-solanine and α-chaconine contents of potatoes. Journal of the Science of Food and Agriculture. 2000;**80**(14):2096-2100. DOI: 10.1002/1097-0010(200011)80:14%3C2096::AID-JSFA757%3E3.0.CO;2-6

[37] Sinden SL, Webb RE. Effect of variety and location on the glycoalkaloid content of potatoes. American Potato Journal. 1972;**49**(9):334-338

[38] Morris SC, Petermann JB. Genetic and environmental effects on levels of glycoalkaloids in cultivars of potato (*Solanum tuberosum* L.). Food Chemistry. 1985;**18**(4):271-282

[39] Levy D, Lisker N, Dimenstein L. The effect of temperature on the content of glycoalkaloids in the tubers. In: Proceedings of the 12th Triennial Conference of EAPR, European Association for Potato Research; Paris; July 1993. pp. 196-197

[40] Roddick JG. Complex formation between *Solanaceous* steroidal

glycoalkaloids and free sterols *in vitro*. Phytochemistry. 1979;**18**(9):1467-1470

[41] Roddick JG. The acetylcholinesterase-inhibitory activity of steroidal glycoalkaloids and their aglycones. Phytochemistry. 1989;**28**(10):2631-2634

[42] Roddick JG, Rijnenberg AL. Effect of steroidal glycoalkaloids of the potato on the permeability of liposome membranes. Physiologia Plantarum. 1986;**68**(3):436-440

[43] Augustin JM, Kuzina V, Andersen SB, Bak S. Molecular activities, biosynthesis and evolution of triterpenoid saponins. Phytochemistry. 2011;**72**(6):435-457. DOI: 10.1016/j.phytochem.2011.01.015

[44] Lin F, Wang R. Hemolytic mechanism of dioscin proposed by molecular dynamics simulations. Journal of Molecular Modeling. 2010;**16**(1):107-118. DOI: 10.1007/s00894-009-0523-0

[45] Langkilde S, Mandimika T, Schrøder M, Meyer O, Slob W, Peijnenburg A, et al. A 28-day repeat dose toxicity study of steroidal glycoalkaloids, α-solanine and α-chaconine in the Syrian Golden hamster. Food and Chemical Toxicology. 2009;**47**(6):1099-1108. DOI: 10.1016/j.fct.2009.01.045

[46] Barceloux DG. Potatoes, tomatoes, and solanine toxicity (*Solanum tuberosum* L., *Solanum lycopersicum* L.). Disease-a-Month. 2009;**55**(6):391-402

[47] Mensinga TT, Sips AJ, Rompelberg CJ, van Twillert K, Meulenbelt J, van den Top HJ, et al. Potato glycoalkaloids and adverse effects in humans: An ascending dose study. Regulatory Toxicology and Pharmacology. 2005;**41**(1):66-72. DOI: 10.1016/j.yrtph.2004.09.004

[48] Patil BC, Sharma RP, Salunkhe DK, Salunkhe K. Evaluation of

solanine toxicity. Food and Cosmetics Toxicology. 1972;**10**(3):395-398

[49] Nishie K, Norred WP, Swain AP. Pharmacology and toxicology of chaconine and tomatine. Research Communications in Chemical Pathology and Pharmacology. 1975;**12**(4):657-668

[50] Blankemeyer JT, White JB, Stringer BK, Friedman M. Effect of α-tomatine and tomatidine on membrane potential of frog embryos and active transport of ions in frog skin. Food and Chemical Toxicology. 1997;**35**(7):639-646. DOI: 10.1016/S0278-6915(97)00038-0

[51] Friedman M, Fitch TE, Yokoyama WE. Lowering of plasma LDL cholesterol in hamsters by the tomato glycoalkaloid tomatine. Food and Chemical Toxicology. 2000;**38**(7):549-553. DOI: 10.1016/S0278-6915(00)00050-8

[52] Valkonen JP, Keskitalo M, Vasara T, Pietilä L, Raman KV. Potato glycoalkaloids: A burden or a blessing? Critical Reviews in Plant Sciences. 1996;**15**(1):1-20

[53] Roddick JG. The steroidal glycoalkaloid α-tomatine. Phytochemistry. 1974;**13**(1):9-25

[54] Zheng X, Xu L, Liang Y, Xiao W, Xie L, Zhang Y, et al. Quantitative determination and pharmacokinetic study of solamargine in rat plasma by liquid chromatography-mass spectrometry. Journal of Pharmaceutical and Biomedical Analysis. 2011;**55**(5):1157-1162. DOI: 10.1016/j.jpba.2011.04.007

[55] Bushway RJ, Bureau JL, King J. Modification of the rapid high-performance liquid chromatographic method for the determination of potato glycoalkaloids. Journal of Agricultural and Food Chemistry. 1986;**34**(2):277-279. DOI: 10.1021/jf00068a032

[56] Bushway RJ, Bureau JL, McGann DF. Alpha-chaconine and alpha-solanine content of potato peels and potato peel products. Journal of Food Science. 1983;**48**(1):84-86. DOI: 10.1111/j.1365-2621.1983.tb14794.x

[57] Mondy NI, Ponnawpalam R. Effect of magnesium fertilizers on total glycoalkaloids and nitrate-N in Katahdin tubers. Journal of Food Science. 1985;**50**(2):535-536. DOI: 10.1111/j.1365-2621.1985.tb13446.x

[58] Machado RM, Toledo MC, Garcia LC. Effect of light and temperature on the formation of glycoalkaloids in potato tubers. Food Control. 2007;**18**(5):503-508. DOI: 10.1016/j.foodcont.2005.12.008

[59] Love SL, Herrman TJ, Thompsonjohns A, Baker TP. Effect and interaction of crop management factors on the glycoalkaloid concentration of potato tubers. Potato Research. 1994;**37**(1):77-85

[60] Salunkhe DK, Wu MT, Jadhav SJ. Effects of light and temperature on the formation of solanine in potato slices. Journal of Food Science. 1972;**37**(6):969-970

[61] Percival G, Dixon G, Sword A. Glycoalkaloid concentration of potato tubers following continuous illumination. Journal of the Science of Food and Agriculture. 1994;**66**(2):139-144

[62] Jadhav SJ, Sharma RP, Salunkhe DK. Naturally occurring toxic alkaloids in foods. CRC Critical Reviews in Toxicology. 1981;**9**(1):21-104

[63] Porter WL. A note on the melting point of α-solanine. American Potato Journal. 1972;**49**(10):403-406

[64] Takagi K, Toyoda M, Fujiyama Y, Saito Y. Effect of cooking on the contents of α-chaconine and α-solanine

in potatoes. Food Hygiene and Safety Science (Shokuhin Eiseigaku Zasshi). 1990;**31**(1):67-73_1

[65] Hoskins FH. Food toxicants, naturally occurring. Kirk-Othmer Encyclopedia of Chemical Technology. 2000:1-23. DOI: 10.1002/0471238961.06 15150408151911.a01.pub2

[66] Uppal DS. Varietal and environmental effect on the glycoalkaloid content of potato (*Solanum tuberosum* L.). Plant Foods for Human Nutrition. 1987;**37**(4): 333-340

[67] Woolfe JA, Poats SV. The Potato in the Human Diet. Cambridge University Press; 1987

[68] Smith DB, Roddick JG, Jones JL. Potato glycoalkaloids: Some unanswered questions. Trends in Food Science and Technology. 1996;7(4):126-131

[69] Kyzlink V, Mikova K, Jelinek R. Tomatine, solanine and embryotoxicity of unripe tomatoes. Sbornik Vysoke skoly chemicko-technologicke v Praze, E: Potraviny. Scientific papers of the Prague Institute of Chemical Technology, E: Food; 1981

[70] Mikova K, Kasova Z, Kyzlink V. Changes in tomatine content in differently preserved tomatoes. Prumysl Potravin. 1981;**32**:196-197

[71] Friedman M, Levin CE. α-Tomatine content in tomato and tomato products determined by HPLC with pulsed amperometric detection. Journal of Agricultural and Food Chemistry. 1995;**43**(6):1507-1511

[72] Lv C, Kong H, Dong G, Liu L, Tong K, Sun H, et al. Antitumor efficacy of α-solanine against pancreatic cancer *in vitro* and *in vivo*. PLoS One. 2014;**9**(2):e87868. DOI: 10.1371/journal. pone.0087868

[73] Friedman M, Lee KR, Kim HJ, Lee IS, Kozukue N. Anticarcinogenic effects of glycoalkaloids from potatoes against human cervical, liver, lymphoma, and stomach cancer cells. Journal of Agricultural and Food Chemistry. 2005;**53**(15):6162-6169. DOI: 10.1021/ jf050620p

[74] Ji YB, Gao SY, Ji CF, Zou X. Induction of apoptosis in HepG2 cells by solanine and Bcl-2 protein. Journal of Ethnopharmacology. 2008;**115**(2):194-202. DOI: 10.1016/j.jep.2007.09.023

[75] Mohsenikia M, Alizadeh AM, Khodayari S, Khodayari H, Karimi A, Zamani M, et al. The protective and therapeutic effects of alpha-solanine on mice breast cancer. European Journal of Pharmacology. 2013;**718**(1-3):1-9. DOI: 10.1016/j.ejphar.2013.09.015

[76] Mohsenikia M, Farhangi B, Alizadeh AM, Khodayari H, Khodayari S, Khori V, et al. Therapeutic effects of dendrosomal solanine on a metastatic breast tumor. Life Sciences. 2016;**148**:260-267. DOI: 10.1016/j. lfs.2016.02.008

[77] Itoh Y, Nagase H. Matrix metalloproteinases in cancer. Essays in Biochemistry. 2002;**38**:21-36

[78] Pan B, Zhong W, Deng Z, Lai C, Chu J, Jiao G, et al. Inhibition of prostate cancer growth by solanine requires the suppression of cell cycle proteins and the activation of ROS/P38 signaling pathway. Cancer Medicine. 2016;**5**(11):3214-3222. DOI: 10.1002/ cam4.916

[79] Lu MK, Shih YW, Chien TT, Fang LH, Huang HC, Chen PS. α-Solanine inhibits human melanoma cell migration and invasion by reducing matrix metalloproteinase-2/9 activities. Biological and Pharmaceutical Bulletin. 2010;**33**(10):1685-1691

[80] Lee KR, Kozukue N, Han JS, Park JH, Chang EY, Baek EJ, et al.

Glycoalkaloids and metabolites inhibit the growth of human colon (HT29) and liver (HepG2) cancer cells. Journal of Agricultural and Food chemistry. 2004;**52**(10):2832-2839. DOI: 10.1021/jf030526d

[81] Ito SI, Ihara T, Tamura H, Tanaka S, Ikeda T, Kajihara H, et al. α-Tomatine, the major saponin in tomato, induces programmed cell death mediated by reactive oxygen species in the fungal pathogen *Fusarium oxysporum*. FEBS Letters. 2007;**581**(17):3217-3222. DOI: 10.1016/j.febslet.2007.06.010

[82] Friedman M, Levin CE, Lee SU, Kim HJ, Lee IS, Byun JO, et al. Tomatine-containing green tomato extracts inhibit growth of human breast, colon, liver, and stomach cancer cells. Journal of Agricultural and Food Chemistry. 2009;**57**(13):5727-5733. DOI: 10.1021/jf900364j

[83] Sucha L, Hroch M, Rezacova M, Rudolf E, Havelek R, Sispera L, et al. The cytotoxic effect of α-tomatine in MCF-7 human adenocarcinoma breast cancer cells depends on its interaction with cholesterol in incubation media and does not involve apoptosis induction. Oncology Reports. 2013;**30**(6):2593-2602. DOI: 10.3892/or.2013.2778

[84] Shieh JM, Cheng TH, Shi MD, Wu PF, Chen Y, Ko SC, et al. α-Tomatine suppresses invasion and migration of human non-small cell lung cancer NCI-H460 cells through inactivating FAK/PI3K/Akt signaling pathway and reducing binding activity of NF-κB. Cell Biochemistry and Biophysics. 2011;**60**(3):297-310. DOI: 10.1007/s12013-011-9152-1

[85] Chao MW, Chen CH, Chang YL, Teng CM, Pan SL. α-Tomatine-mediated anti-cancer activity *in vitro* and *in vivo* through cell cycle-and caspase-independent pathways. PLoS One. 2012;7(9):e44093. DOI: 10.1371/journal.pone.0044093

[86] Rudolf K, Rudolf E. Antiproliferative effects of α-tomatine are associated with different cell death modalities in human colon cancer cells. Journal of Functional Foods. 2016;**27**:491-502. DOI: 10.1016/j.jff.2016.10.005

[87] Huang H, Chen X, Li D, He Y, Li Y, Du Z, et al. Combination of α-tomatine and curcumin inhibits growth and induces apoptosis in human prostate cancer cells. PLoS One. 2015;**10**(12):e0144293. DOI: 10.1371/journal.pone.0144293

[88] Choi SH, Ahn JB, Kozukue N, Kim HJ, Nishitani Y, Zhang L, et al. Structure-activity relationships of α-, β1-, γ-, and δ-tomatine and tomatidine against human breast (MDA-MB-231), gastric (KATO-III), and prostate (PC3) cancer cells. Journal of Agricultural and Food Chemistry. 2012;**60**(15):3891-3899. DOI: 10.1021/jf3003027

[89] Hu K, Kobayashi H, Dong A, Jing Y, Iwasaki S, Yao X. Antineoplastic agents III: Steroidal glycosides from *Solanum nigrum*. Planta Medica. 1999;**65**(01):035-038

[90] Zhou Y, Tang Q, Zhao S, Zhang F, Li L, Wu W, et al. Targeting signal transducer and activator of transcription 3 contributes to the solamargine-inhibited growth and-induced apoptosis of human lung cancer cells. Tumor Biology. 2014;**35**(8):8169-8178. DOI: 10.1007/s13277-014-2047-1

[91] Chen Y, Tang Q, Xiao Q, Yang L, Hann SS. Targeting EP 4 downstream c-Jun through ERK 1/2-mediated reduction of DNMT 1 reveals novel mechanism of solamargine-inhibited growth of lung cancer cells. Journal of Cellular and Molecular Medicine. 2017;**21**(2):222-233. DOI: 10.1111/jcmm.12958

[92] Shiu LY, Chang LC, Liang CH, Huang YS, Sheu HM, Kuo

Food Glycoalkaloids: Distribution, Structure, Cytotoxicity, Extraction, and Biological Activity
DOI: http://dx.doi.org/10.5772/intechopen.82780

KW. Solamargine induces apoptosis and sensitizes breast cancer cells to cisplatin. Food and Chemical Toxicology. 2007;**45**(11):2155-2164. DOI: 10.1016/j.fct.2007.05.009

[93] Sun L, Zhao Y, Li X, Yuan H, Cheng A, Lou H. A lysosomal-mitochondrial death pathway is induced by solamargine in human K562 leukemia cells. Toxicology *in Vitro*. 2010;**24**(6):1504-1511. DOI: 10.1016/j.tiv.2010.07.013

[94] Sun L, Zhao Y, Yuan H, Li X, Cheng A, Lou H. Solamargine, a steroidal alkaloid glycoside, induces oncosis in human K562 leukemia and squamous cell carcinoma KB cells. Cancer Chemotherapy and Pharmacology. 2011;**67**(4):813-821. DOI: 10.1007/s00280-010-1387-9

[95] Ding X, Zhu FS, Li M, Gao SG. Induction of apoptosis in human hepatoma SMMC-7721 cells by solamargine from *Solanum nigrum* L. Journal of Ethnopharmacology. 2012;**139**(2):599-604. DOI: 10.1016/j.jep.2011.11.058

[96] Chang LC, Tsai TR, Wang JJ, Lin CN, Kuo KW. The rhamnose moiety of solamargine plays a crucial role in triggering cell death by apoptosis. Biochemical and Biophysical Research Communications. 1998;**242**(1):21-25. DOI: 10.1006/bbrc.1997.7903

[97] Cham BE. Drug therapy: Solamargine and other solasodine rhamnosyl glycosides as anticancer agents. Modern Chemotherapy. 2013;**2**(02):33

[98] Punjabi S, Cook LJ, Kersey P, Marks R, Cerio R. Solasodine glycoalkaloids: A novel topical therapy for basal cell carcinoma. A double-blind, randomized, placebo-controlled, parallel group, multicenter study. International Journal of

Dermatology. 2008;**47**(1):78-82. DOI: 10.1111/j.1365-4632.2007.03363.x

[99] Roddick JG, Rijnenberg AL. Synergistic interaction between the potato glycoalkaloids α-solanine and α-chaconine in relation to lysis of phospholipid/sterol liposomes. Phytochemistry. 1987;**26**(5):1325-1328

[100] Yamashoji S, Matsuda T. Synergistic cytotoxicity induced by α-solanine and α-chaconine. Food Chemistry. 2013;**141**(2):669-674. DOI: 10.1016/j.foodchem.2013.03.104

[101] Shiu LY, Liang CH, Huang YS, Sheu HM, Kuo KW. Downregulation of HER2/neu receptor by solamargine enhances anticancer drug-mediated cytotoxicity in breast cancer cells with high-expressing HER2/neu. Cell Biology and Toxicology. 2008;**24**(1):1-10. DOI: 10.1007/s10565-007-9010-5

[102] Liang CH, Shiu LY, Chang LC, Sheu HM, Tsai EM, Kuo KW. Solamargine enhances HER2 expression and increases the susceptibility of human lung cancer H661 and H69 cells to trastuzumab and epirubicin. Chemical Research in Toxicology. 2007;**21**(2):393-399. DOI: 10.1021/tx700310x

[103] Shiu LY, Liang CH, Chang LC, Sheu HM, Tsai EM, Kuo KW. Solamargine induces apoptosis and enhances susceptibility to trastuzumab and epirubicin in breast cancer cells with low or high expression levels of HER2/neu. Bioscience Reports. 2009;**29**(1):35-45. DOI: 10.1042/BSR20080028

[104] Chowanski S, Adamski Z, Marciniak P, Rosinski G, Buyukguzel E. A review of bioinsecticidal activity of Solanaceae alkaloids. Toxins. 2016;**8**:60. DOI: 10.3390/toxins8030060, 10.3390/toxins8030060

[105] Friedman M, Huang V, Quiambao Q, Noritake S, Liu J, Kwon O, et al.

Potato peels and their bioactive glycoalkaloids and phenolic compounds inhibit the growth of pathogenic trichomonads. Journal of Agricultural and Food Chemistry. 2018;**66**(30):7942-7947. DOI: 10.1021/acs.jafc.8b01726

[106] Blankemeyer JT, Stringer BK, Rayburn JR, Bantle JA, Friedman M. Effect of potato glycoalkaloids, alpha-chaconine and alpha-solanine on membrane potential of frog embryos. Journal of Agricultural and Food Chemistry. 1992;**40**(10):2022-2025. DOI: 10.1021/jf00022a057

[107] Friedman M, Rayburn JR, Bantle JA. Developmental toxicology of potato alkaloids in the frog embryo teratogenesis assay—Xenopus (FETAX). Food and Chemical Toxicology. 1991;**29**(8):537-547

[108] Rayburn JR, Bantle JA, Friedman M. Role of carbohydrate side chains of potato glycoalkaloids in developmental toxicity. Journal of Agricultural and Food Chemistry. 1994;**42**(7):1511-1515

[109] Fewell AM, Roddick JG. Interactive antifungal activity of the glycoalkaloids α-solanine and α-chaconine. Phytochemistry. 1993;**33**(2):323-328

[110] Fewell AM, Roddick JG, WEIssENBERG MA. Interactions between the glycoalkaloids solasonine and solamargine in relation to inhibition of fungal growth. Phytochemistry. 1994;**37**(4):1007-1011. DOI: 10.1016/S0031-9422(00)89518-7

[111] Fewell AM, Roddick JG. Potato glycoalkaloid impairment of fungal development. Mycological Research. 1997;**101**(5):597-603. DOI: 10.1017/S0953756296002973

[112] Dahlin P, Müller MC, Ekengren S, McKee LS, Bulone V. The impact of steroidal glycoalkaloids on the physiology of *Phytophthora infestans*,

the causative agent of potato late blight. Molecular Plant-Microbe Interactions. 2017;**30**(7):531-542. DOI: 10.1094/MPMI-09-16-0186-R

[113] Nenaah G. Individual and synergistic toxicity of *Solanace*ous glycoalkaloids against two coleopteran stored-product insects. Journal of Pest Science. 2011;**84**(1):77-86. DOI: 10.1007/s10340-010-0329-y

[114] De Sotillo DR, Hadley M, Wolf-Hall C. Potato peel extract a nonmutagenic antioxidant with potential antimicrobial activity. Journal of Food Science. 1998;**63**(5):907-910. DOI: 10.1111/j.1365-2621.1998.tb17924.x

[115] Amanpour R, Abbasi-Maleki S, Neyriz-Naghadehi M, Asadi-Samani M. Antibacterial effects of *Solanum tuberosum* peel ethanol extract *in vitro*. Journal of HerbMed Pharmacology. 2015;**4**

[116] Sandrock RW, VanEtten HD. Fungal sensitivity to and enzymatic degradation of the phytoanticipin α-tomatine. Phytopathology. 1998;**88**(2):137-143. DOI: 10.1094/PHYTO.1998.88.2.137

[117] Ito SI, Eto T, Tanaka S, Yamauchi N, Takahara H, Ikeda T. Tomatidine and lycotetraose, hydrolysis products of α-tomatine by *Fusarium oxysporum* tomatinase, suppress induced defense responses in tomato cells. FEBS Letters. 2004;**571**(1-3):31-34. DOI: 10.1016/j.febslet.2004.06.053

[118] Bouarab K, Melton R, Peart J, Baulcombe D, Osbourn A. A saponin-detoxifying enzyme mediates suppression of plant defences. Nature. 2002;**418**(6900):889. DOI: 10.1038/nature00950

[119] Weissenberg M, Klein M, Meisner J, Ascher KR. Larval growth inhibition of the spiny bollworm, *Earias*

insulana, by some steroidal secondary plant compounds. Entomologia Experimentalis et Applicata. 1986;**42**(3):213-217

[120] Schlösser E. Role of saponins in antifungal resistance. III. Tomatin dependent development of fruit rot organisms on tomato fruits/ Die Rolle von Saponinen im Resistenzmechanismus gegen Pilze. III. Tomatinabhängige Entwicklung von Fruchtfäuleerregern an Tomatenfrüchten. Zeitschrift für Pflanzenkrankheiten und Pflanzenschutz/Journal of Plant Diseases and Protection. 1975:476-484

[121] Liu J, Kanetake S, Wu YH, Tam C, Cheng LW, Land KM, et al. Antiprotozoal effects of the tomato tetrasaccharide glycoalkaloid tomatine and the aglycone tomatidine on mucosal trichomonads. Journal of Agricultural and Food Chemistry. 2016;**64**(46):8806-8810. DOI: 10.1021/acs.jafc.6b04030

[122] Simons V, Morrissey JP, Latijnhouwers M, Csukai M, Cleaver A, Yarrow C, et al. Dual effects of plant steroidal alkaloids on *Saccharomyces cerevisiae*. Antimicrobial Agents and Chemotherapy. 2006;**50**(8):2732-2740. DOI: 10.1128/AAC.00289-06

[123] Fukuhara K, Kubo I. Isolation of steroidal glycoalkaloids from *Solanum incanum* by two countercurrent chromatographic methods. Phytochemistry. 1991;**30**(2):685-687. DOI: 10.1016/0031-9422(91)83753-8

[124] Alzerreca A, Hart G. Molluscicidal steroid glycoalkaloids possessing stereoisomeric spirosolane structures. Toxicology Letters. 1982;**12**(2-3):151-155. DOI: 10.1016/0378-4274(82)90178-3

[125] Thorne HV, Clarke GF, Skuce R. The inactivation of herpes simplex virus by some *Solanaceae* glycoalkaloids. Antiviral Research. 1985;**5**(6):335-343. DOI: 10.1016/0166-3542(85)90003-8

[126] Rowan DD, Macdonald PE, Skipp RA. Antifungal stress metabolites from *Solanum aviculare*. Phytochemistry. 1983;**22**(9):2102-2104

[127] Kusano G, Takahashi A, Sugiyama K, Nozoe S. Antifungal properties of *Solanum* alkaloids. Chemical and Pharmaceutical Bulletin. 1987;**35**(12):4862-4867. DOI: 10.1248/cpb.35.4862

[128] Weissenberg M, Levy A, Svoboda JA, Ishaaya I. The effect of some *Solanum* steroidal alkaloids and glycoalkaloids on larvae of the red flour beetle, *Tribolium castaneum*, and the tobacco hornworm, *Manduca sexta*. Phytochemistry. 1998;**47**(2):203-209. DOI: 10.1016/S0031-9422(97)00565-7

[129] Chataing B, Concepcion JL, Lobaton R, Usubillaga A. Inhibition of *Trypanosoma cruzi* growth *in vitro* by *Solanum* alkaloids: A comparison with ketoconazole. Planta Medica. 1998;**64**:31-36. DOI: 10.1055/s-2006-957361

[130] Choi E, Koo S. Anti-nociceptive and anti-inflammatory effects of the ethanolic extract of potato (*Solanum tuberlosum*). Food and Agricultural Immunology. 2005;**16**(1):29-39. DOI: 10.1080/09540100500064320

[131] Yaksh TL. Spinal systems and pain processing: Development of novel analgesic drugs with mechanistically defined models. Trends in Pharmacological Sciences. 1999;**20**(8):329-337. DOI: 10.1016/S0165-6147(99)01370-X

[132] Kenny OM, McCarthy CM, Brunton NP, Hossain MB, Rai DK, Collins SG, et al. Anti-inflammatory properties of potato glycoalkaloids in stimulated Jurkat and Raw 264.7 mouse macrophages. Life Sciences.

2013;**92**(13):775-782. DOI: 10.1016/j.
lfs.2013.02.006

[133] Shin JS, Lee KG, Lee HH, Lee HJ,
An HJ, Nam JH, et al. α-Solanine isolated
from *Solanum Tuberosum* L. cv Jayoung
abrogates LPS-induced inflammatory
responses via NF-κB inactivation in
RAW 264.7 macrophages and endotoxin-
induced shock model in mice. Journal of
Cellular Biochemistry. 2016;**117**(10):2327-
2339. DOI: 10.1002/jcb.25530

[134] Filderman RB, Kovacs BA. Anti-
inflammatory activity of the steroid
alkaloid glycoside, tomatine.
British Journal of Pharmacology.
1969;**37**(3):748-755

[135] Zhao B, Zhou B, Bao L, Yang
Y, Guo K. Alpha-tomatine exhibits
anti-inflammatory activity in
lipopolysaccharide-activated
macrophages. Inflammation.
2015;**38**(5):1769-1776. DOI: 10.1007/
s10753-015-0154-9

[136] Chiu FL, Lin JK. Tomatidine
inhibits iNOS and COX-2 through
suppression of NF-κB and JNK pathways
in LPS-stimulated mouse macrophages.
FEBS Letters. 2008;**582**(16):2407-2412.
DOI: 10.1016/j.febslet.2008.05.049

[137] Chen Y, Li S, Sun F, Han H, Zhang
X, Fan Y, et al. In vivo antimalarial
activities of glycoalkaloids isolated
from *Solanaceae* plants. Pharmaceutical
Biology. 2010;**48**(9):1018-1024. DOI:
10.3109/13880200903440211

[138] Satoh T. Glycemic effects of
solanine in rats. The Japanese Journal of
Pharmacology. 1967;**17**(4):652-658

[139] Akinnuga AM, Bamidele O,
Ebunlomo AO, Adeniyi OS, Adeleeya
GS, Ebomuche LC. Hypoglycaemic
effects of dietary intake of ripe
and unripe *Lycopersicon esculentum*
[tomatoes] on streptozotocin-induced
diabetes mellitus in rats. On Line Journal
of Biological Sciences. 2010;**10**(2):50-53

Chapter 5

Anti-Corrosive Properties of Alkaloids on Metals

Hui-Jing Li, Weiwei Zhang and Yan-Chao Wu

Abstract

Numerous organic inhibitors have been reported to be used for the corrosion inhibition of various metals, especially, the heterogeneous ring compounds bearing larger electronegativity atoms (i.e., N, O, S, and P), polar functional groups, and conjugated double bonds are the most effective inhibitors. Based on the concept of green chemistry, in recent years, the research of corrosion inhibitor has gradually extracted new environment-friendly corrosion inhibitor from natural animals and plants, because of its advantages in wide source, low cost, low toxicity and subsequent treatment. Alkaloids such as papaverine, strychnine, quinine, nicotine, etc., have been studied as inhibitors for metals corrosion in corrosive media. This chapter aims to review the application of alkaloids for the corrosion inhibition of metals in corrosive media, and the development trend in this field is prospected.

Keywords: iron, steel, copper, aluminum, inhibitor, alkaloids corrosion inhibition

1. Introduction

Metals corrosion is a process in which a metal material loses its basic properties due to the action of the surrounding medium. Despite significant advances in the field of corrosion science and technology, corrosion is still a major obstacle to industry in all countries of the world. Steel, copper, zinc, aluminum as well as their alloys, has been extensively applied in construction and other industrial fields owing to its low price and good material properties [1–4]. However, one of the great challenges that metals face in industrial applications is that they are particularly susceptible to corrosion under acidic or alkaline conditions, which could lead to huge economic losses and potential environmental problems. A practical and cost-effective method to address such problems is the usage of corrosion inhibitors due to their easy synthesis, remarkable inhibition effect and economic advantages. The reported corrosion inhibitors against metals corrosion in acidic or alkaline medium are usually polar organic heterocyclic compounds bearing electronegativity atoms (i.e., nitrogen, oxygen, sulfur, and phosphorus), polar functional groups, and conjugated double bonds [5–7]. For example, azoles [8], Schiff bases [9], quinolones [10], thioureas [11] and pyrimidines [12] have been reported as effective corrosion inhibitors for metals in corrosive medium. The polar units of these corrosion inhibitors are regarded as the reaction centers to promote their adsorption on the metals surface, forming a protective layer to prevent the metals from undertaking corrosion attacks. Nevertheless, corrosion scientists are not very satisfied with chemical inhibitors as they are generally not readily available, expensive, water-insoluble, and pollute the environment in their synthesis and applications processes. With the deterioration of pollution problems, the development and utilization of green, low-toxic organic molecular corrosion inhibitors has received attention. It is highly desirable that the novel metal inhibitors are non-toxic and environmentally friendly.

Recently, the use of natural products as corrosion inhibitors in different media has been widely reported as they are nontoxic, biodegradable and readily available in plenty. Among these natural products, alkaloids (nitrogen as one of their main constituent atoms) such as papaverine, strychnine, quinine, piperine, liriodenine, oxoanalobine and nicotine have been studied as inhibitors for metals corrosion in different media. Moreover, many plants can produce various types of alkaloids which makes this very interesting due to the presence of heteroatoms. These heteroatoms, nitrogen and the oxygen commonly associated with double bonds promote the adsorption between metals and inhibitors [4, 8]. That's why alkaloid plant extracts can reveal the fascinating features about inhibit corrosion, and alkaloids were found to prevent metal corrosion by adsorption of their molecules on metals surface to form a protective layer. Generally, there are two types of interactions of these inhibitors adsorption on metal surface. One is physical adsorption involving the electrostatic force between the ionic charge of the adsorbed species and the charge on the metal surface. The other is chemisorption, which involves charge sharing or transfer from the inhibitor molecules to the metals surface, forming coordination bonds or feedback bonds [9, 13]. Various natural organic inhibitors platforms are needed to develop new cleaning chemicals for green environment, which make the exploitation of late-model alkaloids class of corrosion inhibitors for metal protection a high priority. In this chapter, the corrosion inhibition effects of alkaloids (**Table 1**) as corrosion inhibitors on steel, copper, aluminum and other metal surfaces in different corrosive media such as hydrochloric acid, sulfuric acid, sodium chloride, etc., is reviewed.

2. Alkaloids as corrosion inhibitors

2.1 Iron and steel inhibitor

Iron/steel is a strong metal that is widely used in multitudinous industrial fields, such as machinery manufacturing, petrochemical engineering, constructing and national defensing, etc. The combination of iron and other elements provides many acceptable material properties for application. However, iron materials are highly susceptible to corrosion in acid pickling, acid cleaning, acid descaling and oil well acidification, which will induce potential problems in industrial equipment, consequently leading to huge economic losses and serious environmental pollution. Generally, it is cost-effective to use natural organic inhibitors in acidic media to reduce corrosion of iron and/or steel. It has been reported that the adsorption depends mainly on the electronic and structural properties of the organic inhibitor molecule such as larger electronegativity atoms (i.e., N, O, S, and P), polar functional groups, conjugated double bonds, steric factors, and aromaticity.

Acidic solutions are widely used in various industrial processes, the corrosion and inhibition of iron/steel in this environment constitutes a complex process problem. The use of natural organic inhibitors to reduce the corrosion of iron/steel in acidic media is highly cost-effective, as they are renewable, cheap, easily available and non-toxic. In recent decades, a large number of reports on the inhibition of iron/steel in acid solutions by different types of natural alkaloids inhibitors at

Core moiety	−R	Metal	Medium	References
Berberine	—	Mild steel	1 M H$_2$SO$_4$	[17]
		Copper	0.5 M HCl	[46]
		7075 Al alloy	3.5% NaCl	[57]
		Al alloy	3.5% NaCl	[58]
A: piperine B: piperanine C: pipernonatine	A	Mild steel	1 M HCl	[18]
		C38 steel	1 M HCl	[34]
		Copper	1 M HCl	[47]
	B C	Copper	1 M HCl	[47]
Atheroline	—	Mild steel	1 M HCl	[19] [20]
Brucine	—	Mild steel	1 M HCl	[21]
Caulerpin	—	Mild steel	1 M HCl	[23]
Alstogustine	—	Mild steel	1 M HCl	[24]
Isoreserpiline	—	Mild steel	1 M HCl	[25]

Core moiety	−R	Metal	Medium	References
Isodihydrocadambine	—	Mild steel	1 M HCl	[26]
A: anibine B: 1-(pyridine-2-yl)propan-2-one C: nicotine	A: R$_1$: H and R$_2$:	C38 steel	1 M HCl	[27]
	B: B: R$_1$: and R$_2$: H	Mild steel	8% H$_2$SO$_4$	[41]
	C: R$_1$: H and R$_2$:	Carbon steel	3% NaCl + CO$_2$	[44]
A: isoquinoline B: nornuciferine	A: R$_1$: −CH$_3$ and R$_2$: −OCH$_3$ B: R$_1$: −CH$_3$ and R$_2$: −H	Carbon steel	0.1 M HCl	[30]
Methylmoschatoline	—	Carbon steel	0.1 M HCl	[30]
1-Methyl-pyrido[3,4]indole	—	Carbon steel	0.1 M HCl	[30]
Quinine	—	Carbon steel	1 M HCl	[29]
		Carbon steel	1.5 M HCl	[31]
Dehydrocytisine	—	Carbon steel	1 M HCl	[32]

Core moiety	—R	Metal	Medium	References
 A: cytisine B: methylcytisine C: hydroxylcytisine	A: —H B: —CH$_3$ C: —OH	Carbon steel	1 M HCl	[32]
 A: liriodenine B: oxoanalobine	A: —H B: —OH	C38 steel	1 M HCl	[33]
 Geissospermine	—	C38 steel	1 M HCl	[36]
 A: tryptamine B: indole	A: —(CH$_2$)$_2$NH$_2$ B: —H	Iron Mild steel	0.5 M H$_2$SO$_4$ 1 M HCl 1 M H$_2$SO	[37] [43]
 Brucine	—	Mild steel	1 M H$_2$SO$_4$	[39]
 A: vasicine B: vasicinone	A: —H B: =O	Mild steel	0.5 M H$_2$SO$_4$	[40]
 A: sparteine B: lupanine	A: —H B: =O	Steel 7055-T6 Al alloy Steel 7055-T6 Al alloy	2 M HCl 01 M H$_2$SO$_4$ 0.5 M NaCl 2 M HCl 01 M H$_2$SO$_4$ 0.5 M NaCl	[42] [59] [42] [59]
 Multiflorine	—	Steel 7055-T6 Al alloy	2 M HCl 01 M H$_2$SO$_4$ 0.5 M NaCl	[42] [59]

Core moiety	−R	Metal	Medium	References
 Caffeine	—	Carbon steel	3% NaCl + CO_2	[44]
 Piperidones	R_1: H, R_2: H and R_3: H R_1: H, R_2: −Me and R_3: −Me R_1: −Cl, R_2: H and R_3: H	Copper	0.1 M H_2SO_4	[51]
 2,2-Dimethyl-6-phenylpiperidin-4-one	—	Copper	0.1 M H_2SO_4	[51]
 Emetine	—	Copper	1 M HNO_3	[53]
 Cephaeline	—			

Table 1.
List of alkaloids for corrosion inhibition properties of various metals.

domestic and foreign scholars. As early as the 1970s, the researchers carried out a large number of preliminary exploratory studies on alkaloids corrosion inhibitors, and made some progress. The research of alkaloid corrosion inhibitors is mainly carried out in hydrochloric acid and sulfuric acid medium. In 1986, Ramakrishniah reported an excellent papaverine pickling inhibitor [14], further introducing the research status of alkaloid corrosion inhibitors. It is pointed out that the organic corrosion inhibitor molecule is usually composed of a polar agent centered on N, O atoms and a nonpolar group composed of C, H atoms, which can be bonded with the metal surface in the form of a bond and produce physical or chemical adsorption. Alkaloids namely pyrrolidine [15] as an inhibitor for iron in 1 M HCl; pomegranate [16], berberine [17], piperine [18], atheroline [19, 20], brucine [21], tropane, pyrrolizidine [22], caulerpin [23], indole [24], isoreserpiline [25], 3β-isodihydrocadambine [26], anibine [27], strychnine and quinine [28] as inhibitors for mild steel in 1 M HCl; quinine [29], O-methylisopiline, (−)-nornuciferine, O-methylmoschatoline [30], quinine sulfate (6′-methoxycinchonan-9-ol-sulfate dehydrate) [31] and cytisine [32] as an inhibitor for carbon steel in 1 M HCl; liriodenine, oxoanalobine [33], piperine [34], oxoaporphinoid [35] and geissospermine [36] as inhibitors for C38 steel in 1 M HCl; tryptamine [37] as an inhibitor for iron in 0.5 M H_2SO_4; piperine [38], brucine [39], vasicine, vasicinone [40] and isopelletierine [41] as inhibitors for mild steel in 0.5 M H_2SO_4; sparteine, lupanine, multiflorine [42] and indole [43] as inhibitors for mild steel in 1 M HCl and 0.5 M H_2SO_4 have been investigated against the corrosion of iron/steel by weight loss measurements, potentiodynamic polarization and electrochemical impedance spectroscopy (EIS) techniques. The experimental results revealed that these alkaloids were excellent green inhibitors, and their inhibition efficiency increased with the increase of inhibitor concentration and decreased with increase of temperature. Polarization curve results demonstrate that most of the alkaloids compounds have been classified as mixed inhibitors under the studied acidic conditions. Only the indole alkaloids act as an anodic type inhibitor in HCl and as a mixed type in H_2SO_4 [43]. The Nyquist plots revealed that the charge transfer resistance increased and the double layer capacitance decreased as the concentration of the inhibitor increased. In addition, the inhibition efficiency obtained by weight loss method and electrochemical tests were consistent in all studies. The adsorption of most alkaloids corrosion inhibitors on the steel surface belongs to Langmuir isothermal type. Howbeit, the adsorption of a small amount of alkaloids inhibitors, namely piperine, caulerpin, brucine and quinine on the metal surface was found to obey Temkin's adsorption isotherm in acid medium. But berberine [17] and tryptamine [37] follow the Flory-Huggins adsorption isotherm and Bockris-Swinkels adsorption isotherm on the metal surface, respectively. These adsorption isotherms were calculated from Eqs (1) to (4):

$$\frac{c}{\theta} = \frac{1}{K_{ads}} + c \qquad \text{Langmuir isothermal} \qquad (1)$$

$$\exp(-2a\theta) = K_{ads}c \qquad \text{Temkin's adsorption} \qquad (2)$$

$$\log\left(\frac{\theta}{c}\right) = \log x K_{ads} + x \log(1-\theta) \qquad \text{Flory} - \text{Huggins adsorption} \qquad (3)$$

$$\frac{\theta}{(1-\theta)^x} \frac{[\theta + x(1-\theta)]^{(x-1)}}{x^x} = K_{ads}c \qquad \text{Bockris} - \text{Swinkels adsorption} \qquad (4)$$

where c is inhibitor concentration, θ represents surface coverage, x means the number of adsorbed water molecules replaced by one inhibitor molecule. The formation and properties of the adsorbed films on the steel surface have been investigated using scanning electron microscope (SEM) [17, 19, 20, 22, 24–26, 36, 38, 39, 43], X-ray photoelectron spectroscopy (XPS) [27, 32], FTIR spectroscopy [19–26, 39, 41, 43] and atomic force microscopy (AFM) [23]. The effect of temperature on inhibitive performances were studied to provide more detailed insights into the kinetics and thermodynamics of metal corrosion in acid solutions. Quantum chemical calculations were employed to provide insightful quantitative information to conclude the correlation between molecular structures and inhibition performance.

Metal corrosion also occurs in industrial processes under neutral conditions. Therefore, inhibiting metal corrosion under neutral conditions is also an important research direction. Numerous studies revealed that caffeine and nicotine can act as effective corrosion inhibitors for iron/steel in neutral environment. Corrosion inhibition of carbon steel by caffeine (1,3,7-trimethyl-purine-2,6-dione) and nicotine (3-(1-methylpyrrolidin-2-yl)pyridine) [44] in 3% NaCl solution with CO_2 was investigated using various techniques. Potentiodynamic polarization curve results showed that these compounds belonged to mixed-type inhibitors which primarily inhibited the cathodic reaction, and this effect still exists at low inhibitor concentration, indicating that these compounds are good inhibitors in 3% NaCl + CO_2 conditions ($\eta > 90\%$ for caffeine and > 80% for nicotine). The thermodynamic analysis of Langmuir model shows that the adsorption of these alkaloids is physical adsorption. Surface analysis (SEM-EDS) confirmed that the inhibition effect was due to the adsorption of caffeine or nicotine molecules on the surface of carbon steel solution. The effect of temperature for caffeine and nicotine was also studied by electrochemical impedance spectroscopy (EIS), demonstrating that the best inhibitor was caffeine, as its structure has more active sites in the oxygen and nitrogen heteroatoms, and more easily adsorbed on the steel surface. In addition, caffeine (1,3,7-trimethylamine) and nicotine (1-methyl-2-pyrrolidinyl) pyridine) [45] as corrosion inhibitors for cast iron in 0.1 M Na_2SO_4 solution was evaluated by electrochemical techniques. The results showed that the two compounds added as corrosion inhibitors showed considerable corrosion resistance. The formation of bimolecular layer by additives can effectively inhibit oxidation and improve the protection performance of WD-40 oil.

2.2 Copper inhibitor

Copper and its alloys have a wide range of applications in the industrial field due to their high electrical and thermal conductivity. Nevertheless, copper is extremely sensitive to corrosion in acid and alkaline solutions, and thus result in huge economic losses and potential environmental problems. A practical and effective solution to this problem is to use organic corrosion inhibitors. At present, the copper corrosion inhibitors used in industry mainly include: azole type, amine type and pyridine type corrosion inhibitors mainly containing N compounds. However, such compounds are highly toxic and pose a great hazard to operators and the environment. Therefore, the research and development of high efficiency, low toxicity, environment-friendly corrosion inhibitor is one of the main directions of corrosion inhibitor development. In recent years, researchers have applied natural alkaloids as copper corrosion inhibitors, which are non-toxic, environmentally friendly, simple preparation process and low cost. These organic compounds customarily contain polar functional groups with N, S or O atoms, and have triple or conjugated double bonds in their molecular structure, which are the main adsorption centers.

The research on the inhibition effect of alkaloids on copper is mainly carried out in hydrochloric acid, sulfuric acid and nitric acid. Corrosion inhibition of copper by berberine (5,6-dihydro-9,10-dimethoxybenzo[g]-1,3-benzodioxolo[5,6-a] quinoliziniu-m) [46] in 0.5 M HCl and piperine, piperanine, pipernonatine, N-11-(3,4-methyl-enedioxyphenylhmdecatrienoyl)-piperidine [47] in 1 M HCl; caffeine [48], quinine, strychnine [49, 50], piperidine, piperidones (2,6-diphcnylpiperidin-4-on, 3-methyl-2,6-diphenylpiperidin-4-on, 2,2-dimethyl-6-phenylpiperidin-4-one, N-chloro-2-6-diphenylpiperidin-4-on) [51] in 0.1 M H_2SO_4; hyoscine, atropine, hyoscyamine [52], emetine, cephaeline [53] in 1 M HNO_3 was investigated by gravimetric, electrochemical, surface, and quantum chemical calculations methods. These compounds were found to exhibit good inhibition performance and the corrosion inhibition efficiency increased with increasing concentration. Polarization curves showed that all of those alkaloids are determined as mixed-type inhibitors in the studied solutions, and the results were consistent with those obtained by weight loss. The adsorption of a majority of alkaloids on copper surface obeys the Langmuir isotherm model, whereas quinine and strychnine were found to follow Bockris-Swinkels adsorption isotherm in 0.1 M H_2SO_4 solution. The surface morphologies of copper specimens after immersion in test solution without and with studied alkaloids inhibitors were observed by SEM and AFM. These experimental results were also supported by quantum chemical calculations, which provided insightful quantitative information to conclude the correlation between molecular structures and inhibition performance.

Besides, copper can be severely corroded in sea water and chloride environments due to the presence of large amounts of chloride ions, and the anodic dissolution of copper is affected by the concentration of chloride ions. When the chloride ion concentration is below 1 M, the anode dissolves to form CuCl, followed by the formation of $CuCl_2$ when excess chloride ions are present [54]. The inhibition effect of some alkaloids on copper has been evaluated by various techniques. For example, see [14] papaverine, brucine, strychnine, ephedrine and cinchonidine was investigated using weight loss in 100 ppm sodium chloride solutions. It's interesting to note that brucine, strychnine and cinchonidine can inhibit the corrosion of copper, while papaverine and ephedrine accelerate the corrosion of copper. The results also showed that cinchonidine had the best inhibition performance with an efficiency of 94%. In addition, the corrosion inhibitive action of copper corrosion in 1.5% sodium chloride solution was studied by various forms of the piperidine moiety [55]. Results indicated that both piperidine and piperidine dithiocarbamate were excellent copper corrosion inhibitors, and the properties of two compounds are classified as mixed-type inhibitors. At the optimum concentration, the maximum inhibition efficiency of the two compounds differs significantly, which is mainly determined by the properties of the substituents in the molecule. These studies have shown that the adsorption of corrosion inhibitor on the copper surface to form a protective film is the main reason for inhibiting copper corrosion. The adsorbed alkaloid forms a complex with Cu^+, thereby preventing the formation of copper chloride complexes.

2.3 Aluminum and their alloys inhibitor

Aluminum and its alloys are widely used in aviation, construction and automotive industries due to their light, good electrical and thermal conductivity, high reflectivity, high strength-to-density ratio and oxidation resistance. The oxidation layer of aluminum has a natural corrosion protection, but if exposed to an erosive environment, the metal is highly susceptible to corrosion, especially in the presence of chloride ions (Cl^-), such as in seawater and sodium chloride solution, the oxide is broken down. Therefore, it is still a great challenge to improve the corrosion resistance of aluminum and its alloys. Corrosion inhibitors are widely used in the industry to reduce the corrosion rate of metals and alloys in contact with corrosive environments.

Some literature studies have shown that various alkaloid corrosion inhibitors are widely used to prevent the dissolution of aluminum and its alloys in alkaline and chloride solution. The corrosion inhibition of pyridine for aluminum in 1 M NaOH solution [56], berberine namely 5,6-dihydro-9,10-dimethoxybenzo[g]-1,3-benzodioxolo[5,6-a]quinolizinium for 7075 aluminum alloy in 3.5% NaCl solution [57, 58], sparteine, lupanine and multiflorine for 7075-T6 aluminum alloy in 0.5 M NaCl solution [59] has been evaluated by weight loss, potentiodynamic polarization and EIS techniques. It is found that they are mixed type inhibitors in the studied conditions. In addition to the Temkin's adsorption of 5,6-dihydro-9,10-dimethoxybenzo[g]-1,3-benzodioxolo[5,6-a]quinolizinium, the adsorption of other alkaloids inhibitor on the copper surface follows Langmuir adsorption isothermal type. The thermodynamic parameters such as free energy, adsorption enthalpy, entropy and activation parameters were calculated to study the adsorption mechanism. In some alkaloid studies, SEM, SECM, UV were implemented to investigate the correlation between the surface properties of metals and electrochemical corrosion behavior, and the adsorption behaviors of molecules on the aluminum and its alloys surface was discussed by electrochemical test and surface analysis.

3. Development prospect

With the progress and development of industry and science and technology, the corrosion inhibitor science and technology has been developed and improved, and the researchers have done a lot of work on the research direction of inhibitors. Among them, environment-friendly corrosion inhibitors, especially alkaloids, have aroused wide attention of researchers and become one of the main directions of the development of corrosion inhibitors in the future. Despite the progress and achievements in the study of alkaloids corrosion inhibitors, there are still many problems that need to be solved. There are many varieties of alkaloids corrosion inhibitors developed by researchers, but not many industrialized production, which is mainly due to the large amount of alkaloid inhibitors and high cost compared with the corrosion inhibitors currently used in industry. Therefore, in the future, we should focus on the study of extracting effective constituents from natural plants, marine flora and fauna, and strengthening the study of low toxicity or non-toxic organic molecule corrosion inhibitor synthesized by synthetic multifunctional base, and making the corrosion inhibitor by compounding or modifying to realize the optimum utilization of resources. In addition, the theory is imperfect, the molecular design lacks the theory instruction. Molecular design has been widely used in the development of fine chemicals, but in the development of environmentally friendly corrosion inhibitor new products due to the lack of systematic theoretical guidance, there is still controversy over the mechanism of corrosion inhibition of many corrosion inhibitors. This requires the use of advanced chemical technologies such as quantum chemistry theory and molecular design to synthesize efficient, multifunctional and environmentally friendly organic corrosion inhibitors. At the same time, using modern advanced analytical instruments and computers to study the adsorption behavior and mechanism of inhibitor molecules on metal surface from the molecular and atomic levels to guide the research and development of corrosion inhibitors.

4. Conclusions

The corrosion inhibition effects of alkaloids on different metals in various corrosion media at room and higher temperature was reviewed. Weight loss, electrochemical studies, surface morphology and quantum chemical studies have been reviewed. The inhibition behavior of alkaloid inhibitors on metals was reviewed by weight loss method, electrochemical measurements, surface analysis and quantum chemical calculations. The studies showed that all these alkaloids are good corrosion inhibitors and the majority alkaloids acted as mixed-type inhibitor. Various adsorption isotherms were analyzed, the majority alkaloids were found to follow the Langmuir adsorption isotherm, and a few followed Bockris-Swinkels and Temkin's adsorption. This review will be useful for corrosion inhibitor research and provide new possible considerations in the design of practical alkaloids-type corrosion inhibitors for metals in corrosive solution.

Acknowledgements

This work was supported by the National Natural Science Foundation of China (21672046, 21372054), the Fundamental Research Funds for the Central Universities (HIT.NSRIF.201701), and the Science and Technology Development Project of Weihai (2012DXGJ02, 2015DXGJ04).

Conflict of interest

On behalf of all authors, the corresponding author states that there is no conflict of interest.

Author details

Hui-Jing Li*, Weiwei Zhang and Yan-Chao Wu
School of Marine Science and Technology, Harbin Institute of Technology, Weihai, P.R. China

*Address all correspondence to: lihuijing@iccas.ac.cn

IntechOpen

References

[1] Zhang WW, Li HJ, Wang YW, Liu Y, Gu QZ, Wu YC. Gravimetric, electrochemical and surface studies on the anticorrosive properties of 1-(2-pyridyl)-2-thiourea and 2-(imidazol-2-yl)-pyridine for mild steel in hydrochloric acid. New Journal of Chemistry. 2018;**42**:12649-12665

[2] Husain E, Narayanan TN, Taha-Tijerina JJ, Vinod S, Vajtai R, Ajayan PM. Marine corrosion protective coatings of hexagonal boron nitride thin films on stainless steel. ACS Applied Materials & Interfaces. 2013;**5**: 4129-4135

[3] Singh P, Srivastava V, Quraishi MA. Novel quinoline derivatives as green corrosion inhibitors for mild steel in acidic medium: Electrochemical, SEM, AFM, and XPS studies. Journal of Molecular Liquids. 2016;**216**:164-173

[4] Zhang WW, Ma R, Li S, Liu Y, Niu L. Electrochemical and quantum chemical studies of azoles as corrosion inhibitors for mild steel in hydrochloric acid. Chemical Research in Chinese Universities. 2016;**32**:827-837

[5] Verma C, Olasunkanmi LO, Ebenso EE, Quraishi MA. 2,4-Diamino-5-(phenylthio)-5H-chromeno [2,3-b] pyridine-3-carbonitriles as green and effective corrosion inhibitors: Gravimetric, electrochemical, surface morphology and theoretical studies. RSC Advances. 2016;**6**:53933-53948

[6] Olasunkanmi LO, Obot IB, Kabanda MM, Ebenso EE. Some quinoxalin-6-yl derivatives as corrosion inhibitors for mild steel in hydrochloric acid: Experimental and theoretical studies. Journal of Physical Chemistry C. 2015; **119**:16004-16019

[7] Elmsellem H, Basbas N, Chetouani A, Aouniti A, Radi S, Messali M, et al. Quantum chemical studies and corrosion inhibitive properties of mild steel by some pyridine derivatives in 1 N HCl solution. Portugaliae Electrochimica Acta. 2014;**32**:77-108

[8] Aljourani J, Raeissi K, Golozar MA. Benzimidazole and its derivatives as corrosion inhibitors for mild steel in 1 M HCl solution. Corrosion Science. 2009; **51**:1836-1843

[9] Behpour M, Ghoreishi SM, Mohammadi N, Soltani N, Salavati-Niasaria M. Investigation some schiff base compounds containing disulfide bonds as HCl corrosion inhibitors for mild steel. Corrosion Science. 2010;**52**: 4046-4057

[10] Zhang WW, Ma R, Liu HH, Liu Y, Li S, Niu L. Electrochemical and surface analysis studies of 2-(quinolin-2-yl) quinazolin-4(3H)-one as corrosion inhibitor for Q235 steel in hydrochloric acid. Journal of Molecular Liquids. 2016; **222**:671-679

[11] Li X, Deng S, Fu H. Allyl thiourea as a corrosion inhibitor for cold rolled steel in H₃PO₄ solution. Corrosion Science. 2012;**52**:280-288

[12] Li X, Xue X, Deng S, Du G. Two phenylpyrimidine derivatives as new corrosion inhibitors for cold rolled steel in hydrochloric acid solution. Corrosion Science. 2014;**87**:27-39

[13] Zhang WW, Li HJ, Wang YW, Liu Y, Wu YC. Adsorption and corrosion inhibition properties of pyridine-2-aldehyde-2-quinolylhydrazone for Q235 steel in acid medium: Electrochemical, thermodynamic, and surface studies. Materials and Corrosion

[14] Ramakrishniah K. Role of some biologically important compounds on the corrosion of mild steel and copper in

sodium chloride solutions. Bulletin of Electrochemistry. 1986;**2**:7-10

[15] Hammouti B, Kertit S, Melhaoui A. Bgugaine: A natural pyrrolidine alkaloid product as corrosion inhibitor of iron in acid chloride solution. Bulletin of Electrochemistry. 1995;**11**:553

[16] Jha LJ, Hussain A, Singh G. Pomegranate alkaloids as corrosion inhibitor for mild steel in acidic medium. Journal of the Electrochemical Society of India. 1991;**40**:153-160

[17] Li Y, Zhao P, Liang Q, Hou BR. Berberine as a natural source inhibitor for mild steel in 1 M H_2SO_4. Applied Surface Science. 2005;**252**:1245-1253

[18] Quraishi MA, Yadav DK, Ahamad I. Green approach to corrosion inhibition by black pepper extract in hydrochloric acid solution. The Open Corrosion Journal. 2009;**2**:56-60

[19] Raja PB, Rahim AA, Osman H, Awang K. Inhibitive effect of Xylopia ferruginea extract on the corrosion of mild steel in 1 M HCl medium. International Journal of Minerals, Metallurgy, and Materials. 2011;**18**: 413-418

[20] Elyn Amira WAW, Rahim AA, Osman H, Awang K, Bothi Raja P. Corrosion inhibition of mild steel in 1 M HCl solution by Xylopia ferruginea leaves from different extract and partitions. International Journal of Electrochemical Science. 2011;**6**: 2998-3016

[21] Singh A, Singh VK, Quraishi MA. Inhibition effect of environmentally benign Kuchla (Strychnos nuxvomica) seed extract on corrosion of mild steel in hydrochloric acid solution. Rasayan Journal of Chemistry. 2010;**3**:811-824

[22] Gopiraman M, Sakunthala P, Kesavan D, Alexramani V, Kim IS, Sulochana N. An investigation of mild

carbon steel corrosion inhibition in hydrochloric acid medium by environment friendly green inhibitors. Journal of Coating Technology and Research. 2012;**9**:15-26

[23] Kamal C, Sethuraman MG. Caulerpin-A bis-indole alkaloid as a green inhibitor for the corrosion of mild steel in 1 M HCl solution from the marine alga caulerpa racemose. Industrial and Engineering Chemistry Research. 2012;**51**:10399-10407

[24] Raja PB, Qureshi AK, Rahim AA, Awang K, Mukhtar MR, Osman H. Indole alkaloids of alstonia angustifolia var. latifolia as green inhibitor for mild steel corrosion in 1 M HCl media. Journal of Materials Engineering and Performance. 2013;**22**:1072-1078

[25] Raja PB, Fadaeinasab M, Qureshi AK, Rahim AA, Osman H, Litaudon M, et al. Evaluation of green corrosion inhibition by alkaloid extracts of ochrosia oppositifolia and isoreserpiline against mild steel in 1 M HCl medium. Industrial and Engineering Chemistry Research. 2013;**52**:10582-10593

[26] Raja PB, Qureshi AK, Rahim AA, Osman H, Awang K. Neolamarckia cadamba alkaloids as eco-friendly corrosion inhibitors for mild steel in 1 M HCl media. Corrosion Science. 2013;**69**: 292-301

[27] Chevalier M, Robert F, Amusant N, Traisnel M, Roos C, Lebrini M. Enhanced corrosion resistance of mild steel in 1 M hydrochloric acid solution by alkaloids extract from Aniba rosaeodora plant: Electrochemical, phytochemical and XPS studies. Electrochimica Acta. 2014;**131**:96-105

[28] Alagbe M. Mechanism investigations of corrosion inhibition of NST-44 mild steel in 1 M hydrochloric acid by caffeine strychnine and quinine. International Conference of Science, Engineering and Environmental Technology. 2017;**2**:16-22

[29] Awad MI. Eco friendly corrosion inhibitors: Inhibitive action of quinine for corrosion of low carbon steel in 1 m HCl. Journal of Applied Electrochemistry. 2006;**36**:1163-1168

[30] Lecante A, Robert F, Blandinières PA, Roos C. Anti-corrosive properties of S. tinctoria and G. ouregou alkaloid extracts on low carbon steel. Current Applied Physics. 2011;**11**:714-724

[31] Samide A, Tutunaru B. Quinine sulfate: A pharmaceutical product as effective corrosion inhibitor for carbon steel in hydrochloric acid solution. Central European Journal of Chemistry. 2014;**12**:901-908

[32] El Hamdani N, Fdil R, Tourabi M, Jama C, Bentiss F. Alkaloids extract of Retama monosperma (L.) Boiss. Seeds used as novel eco-friendly inhibitor for carbon steel corrosion in 1 M HCl solution: Electrochemical and surface studies. Applied Surface Science. 2015;**357**:1294-1305

[33] Lebrini M, Robert F, Roos C. Inhibition effect of alkaloids extract from annona squamosa plant on the corrosion of C38 steel in normal hydrochloric acid medium. International Journal of Electrochemical Science. 2010;**5**:1698-1712

[34] Dahmani M, Et-Touhami A, Al-Deyab SS, Hammouti B, Bouyanzer A. Corrosion inhibition of C38 steel in 1 M HCl: A comparative study of black pepper extract and its isolated piperine. International Journal of Electrochemical Science. 2010;**5**:1060-1069

[35] Lebrini M, Robert F, Lecante A, Roos C. Corrosion inhibition of C38 steel in 1 M hydrochloric acid medium by alkaloids extract from Oxandra asbeckii plant. Corrosion Science. 2011;**53**:687-695

[36] Faustin M, Maciuk A, Salvin P, Roos C, Lebrini M. Corrosion inhibition of C38 steel by alkaloids extract of Geissospermum laeve in 1 M hydrochloric acid: Electrochemical and phytochemical studies. Corrosion Science. 2015;**92**:287-300

[37] Moretti G, Guidi F, Grion G. Tryptamine as a green iron corrosion inhibitor in 0.5 M deaerated sulphuric acid. Corrosion Science. 2004;**46**: 387-403

[38] Bothi Raja P, Sethuraman MG. Inhibitive effect of black pepper extract on the sulphuric acid corrosion of mild steel. Materials Letters. 2008;**62**: 2977-2979

[39] Bothi Raja P, Sethuraman MG. Strychnos nux-vomica an eco-friendly corrosion inhibitor for mild steel in 1 M sulfuric acid medium. Materials and Corrosion. 2009;**60**:22-27

[40] Ramananda Singh M. A green approach: A corrosion inhibition of mild steel by adhatoda vasica plant extract in 0.5 M H_2SO_4. Journal of Materials and Environmental Science. 2013;**4**:119-126

[41] Saxena A, Prasad D, Haldhar R. Withania somnifera extract as green inhibitor for mild steel in 8% H_2SO_4. Asian Journal of Chemistry. 2016;**28**: 2471-2474

[42] Abdel-Gaber AM, Abd-El-Nabey BA, Saadawy M. The role of acid anion on the inhibition of the acidic corrosion of steel by lupine extract. Corrosion Science. 2009;**51**:1038-1042

[43] Pandian Bothi R, Afidah Abdul R, Hasnah O, Khalijah A. Inhibitory effect of kopsia singapurensis extract on the corrosion behavior of mild steel in acid media. Acta Physico-Chimica Sinica. 2010;**26**:2171-2176

[44] Espinoza-Vazquez A, Rodríguez-Gómez FJ. Caffeine and nicotine in 3% NaCl solution with CO_2 as corrosion

inhibitors for low carbon steel. RSC Advances. 2016;**6**:70226-70236

[45] Roncagliolo-Barrera P, Rodríguez-Gómez FJ. Electrochemical evaluation of WD-40 oil as temporary protection with additions of natural compounds as inhibitors in cast iron. ECS Transactions. 2018;**84**:139-147

[46] Karadas N, Akbas A. Inhibition effect of berberine on the corrosion of copper in acidic medium. Revue Roumaine de Chimie. 2013;**58**:639-645

[47] Cai L, Fu Q, Shi RW, Tang Y, Long YT, He XP, et al. 'Pungent' copper surface resists acid corrosion in strong HCl solutions. Industrial and Engineering Chemistry Research. 2014;**53**:64-69

[48] Ahmed MF, Mayanna SM, Pushpanaden F. Effect of caffeine on the anodic dissolution of copper (100) plane in acidic copper sulfate solution. Journal of the Electrochemical Society. 1977;**124**:1667-1671

[49] Subramanyam NC, Sheshadri BC, Mayanna SM. Quinine and strychnine as corrosion inhibitors for copper in sulphuric acid. British Corrosion Journal. 1984;**19**:177-180

[50] Nandeesh LS, Sheshadri BS. The anisotropic nature of copper corrosion and inhibition in sulphuric acid containing strychnine. Corrosion Science. 1988;**28**:19-32

[51] Sankarapapavinasam S, Pushpanaden F, Ahmed MF. Piperidine, piperidones and tetrahydrothiopyrones as inhibitors for the corrosion of copper in H_2SO_4. Corrosion Science. 1991;**32**:193-203

[52] Fouda AS, Abdallah YM, Elawady GY, Ahmed RM. Electrochemical study on the effectively of Hyoscyamus Muticus extract as a green inhibitor for corrosion of copper in 1 M HNO_3.

Journal of Materials and Environmental Science. 2015;**5**:1519-1531

[53] Younis RM, Hassan HM, Mansour RA, El-desoky AM. Corrosion inhibition of carapichea ipecacuanha extract (CIE) on copper in 1 M HNO_3 solution. International Journal of Scientific and Engineering Research. 2015;**6**:761-770

[54] Phadke Swathi N, Alva VPD, Samshuddin S. A review on 1,2,4-Triazole derivatives as corrosion inhibitors. Journal of Bio- and Tribo-Corrosion. 2017;**3**:42-53

[55] Singh MM, Rastogi RB, Upadhyay BN. Inhibition of copper corrosion in aqueous sodium chloride solution by various forms of the piperidine moiety. Corrosion. 1994;**50**:620-625

[56] Singh A, Ahamad I, Quraishi MA. Piper longum extract as green corrosion inhibitor for aluminium in NaOH solution. Arabian Journal of Chemistry. 2016;**9**:1584-1589

[57] Singh A, Lin YH, Liu WY, Yu SJ, Pan J, Ren CQ, et al. Plant derived cationic dye as an effective corrosion inhibitor for 7075 aluminum alloy in 3.5% NaCl solution. Journal of Industrial and Engineering Chemistry. 2014;**20**:4276-4285

[58] Liu WY, Singh A, Lin YH, Ebenso EE, Guan TH, Ren CQ. Corrosion inhibition of Al-alloy in 3.5% NaCl solution by a natural inhibitor: An electrochemical and surface study. International Journal of Electrochemical Science. 2014;**9**:5560-5573

[59] Fetouh HA, Abdel-Fattah TM, El-Tantawy MS. Novel plant extracts as green corrosion inhibitors for 7075-T6 aluminium alloy in an aqueous medium. International Journal of Electrochemical Science. 2014;**9**:1565-1582

www.ingramcontent.com/pod-product-compliance
Lightning Source LLC
Chambersburg PA
CBHW070241230326
41458CB00100B/5760